Obstetrical Casebooks of Dr. Ferdinand E. Chatard

An Alternative
Genealogical Resource for
Baltimore City, Maryland
1829-1883

Gary B. Ruppert, M.D

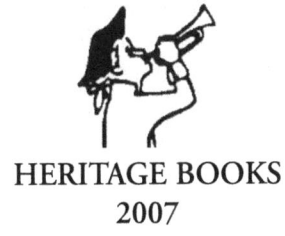

HERITAGE BOOKS
2007

HERITAGE BOOKS
AN IMPRINT OF HERITAGE BOOKS, INC.

Books, CDs, and more—Worldwide

For our listing of thousands of titles see our website
at
www.HeritageBooks.com

Published 2007 by
HERITAGE BOOKS, INC.
Publishing Division
65 East Main Street
Westminster, Maryland 21157-5026

Copyright © 2007 Gary B. Ruppert, M.D.

Other books by the author:

Index to Baptisms, Burials and Confirmations, Second German Evangelical Lutheran Church, Baltimore City, Maryland, 1835-1867

Trinity Lutheran Church Records: Baltimore, Maryland

All rights reserved. No part of this book may be reproduced or transmitted in any form or by any means, electronic or mechanical, including photocopying, recording or by any information storage and retrieval system without written permission from the author, except for the inclusion of brief quotations in a review.

International Standard Book Number: 978-0-7884-4331-3

Acknowledgements

Genealogists are always on the watch for unique resources. At the inaugural Spring Luncheon of the Maryland Genealogical Society in 2004, Nancy Bramucci presented, "Maryland Medical Care in the Nineteenth-Century, A Guide for Genealogists." She mentioned that the Medical and Chirurgical Faculty of Maryland had recently transferred much of their historic records collection to the Maryland Historical Society. Later in an e-mail she provided the reference to Dr. Ferdinand Edme Chatard's case books that ultimately led to my transcription.

The staff of Special Collections at the Maryland Historical Society Library has been very cooperative in pulling the appropriate records and collections for my review. Furthermore, they have very kindly kept the records readily available for my access. Thanks go to Elisabeth Proffen, David Angerhofer, Jim Emmons and Joe Tropea.

Debra Sciabarrasi of MedChi in Baltimore was very kind to give me a personal tour of the Society's collection of paintings and sculptures of what she described as "our dead white men." The beautiful painting of Dr. Ferdinand E. Chatard (depicted on the cover) was found hanging in MedChi's Osler Hall.

Gary B. Ruppert, MD
August 2006

Obstetrical Casebooks of Dr. Ferdinand E. Chatard, 1829-1883

Pierre Chatard established the groundwork of a five-generation medical dynasty in Maryland when he settled in Baltimore Town in 1800. Pierre and his son Ferdinand Edme maintained detailed obstetrical records including names, dates, and number of prior children, occasionally an age or address and always medical details about the woman's "confinement."

When the Medical and Chirurgical Faculty of Maryland transferred historical manuscripts from their library to the Maryland Historical Society, many artifacts of the Chatard family were included. Among this collection are five volumes of handwritten notes concerning deliveries of women in Baltimore City from 1828 through 1883. These include two volumes by Pierre Chatard (covering the years 1828-1846) and three volumes from Ferdinand E. Chatard (covering the years 1829-1883).

Since civil birth registration did not commence in Baltimore until 1875, the Chatard obstetrical volumes represent a remarkable resource for genealogists. Not only do they include the mother's name, date of birth of the child and the child's gender, but often there are extensive personal details not only about the medical aspects of the pregnancy but also about the woman. As a physician, the details of this nineteenth-century medical care have been especially interesting to me. There are numerous mentions of cupping and bleeding not to overlook the application of brandy, use of opium as well as introduction of chloroform.

Obstetrical Casebooks of Dr. F. E. Chatard

Dr. Chatard also describes the use of various types of obstetrical forceps.

The Chatard Family

Pierre Chatard was the first of five generations of Chatard physicians all of whom have lived and practiced in Maryland. The Chatard family history is interesting as it encompasses moves from France to the French West Indies to Delaware and to Maryland.[1]

Pierre Chatard was born in July 1766 in Cape Francois, Dominican Republic. He was the son of Pierre Chatard born in St. Yrieix in Limousin, France. The family immigrated to Domincan Republic in the French West Indies where they owned a coffee plantation. Pierre Chatard, the son was educated in France earning an undergraduate degree in 1785 in Toulouse. In 1788 he had obtained a medical degree from the medical school at Montpelier following which he returned to Santo Domingo but subsequently sought further surgical training in Paris. While in Paris, revolution broke out among the slaves on the West Indies Island and his parents and family fled to Delaware. Dr. Chatard joined them in Wilmington in 1794 where he began his medical practice. After the deaths of his parents in 1797, he returned to claim the family estate in the Caribbean. By May 1800, he feared further uprisings and fled on the ship *Sympathy* only to be captured by the British. He was transferred to the schooner *Elizabeth*. With permission of the British

---

[1] All of the family data were extracted from Dixie Walker Young's *Chatard Family Journal* published during the 1970s.

Alternative Genealogical Source 1829-1883

captain, Dr. Chatard was allowed to sail to Baltimore, which was the homeport for the schooner. It was there that he settled remained for the duration of his life.

On 28 October 1801, Pierre Chatard married in Baltimore's Catholic Cathedral (known then as St. Peter's) to Jeanne Marie Adelaide Francoise Boisson who had also been born at Cape Francois and was educated in France. Dr. Chatard died in Baltimore on 5 June 1848. Children of Pierre Chatard and Jeanne M. A. F. Boisson are as follows:

1. Jane Louise Helen Chatard 21 October 1802 – 6 September 1803
2. Peter Francis Henry Chatard 5 June 1804-20 December 1823
3. Ferdinand Edme Chatard 3 August 1805-18 October 1888
4. Frederick Peter Chatard 17 May 1807-3 October 1897 married (1) Catherine J. Tiernan and (2) Elise McNally. Frederick was a commander in the United States Navy but joined the Confederacy during the Civil War. After the war he settled in St. Louis, Missouri where he died at age 90.
5. Mary Amalie or Emily Chatard 24 November 1808-2 January 1879 married to Frederick J. Dugan
6. un-named infant Chatard died 1813
7. Joseph Mark Auguste Chatard 20 October 1815-17 August 1817
8. Joseph Francis Chatard 1 July 1818-23 September 1835

Obstetrical Casebooks of Dr. F. E. Chatard

9. Mary Josephine Chatard 13 July 1821-23 January 1903 married Chew Van Bibber

Ferdinand Edme Chatard, son of Pierre and Jeanne M. A. F. Boisson Chatard was born in Baltimore City on 3 August 1805. His undergraduate education was completed at Mount St. Mary's College in Emmittsburg, Frederick County, Maryland as well as at St. Mary's in Baltimore. He studied in Baltimore City obtaining his medical degree in 1826 from the College of Physicians and Surgeons (affiliated with the University of Maryland School of Medicine). Following graduation he studied in France for three years obtaining further medical skills after which he returned to Baltimore where he began medical practice in 1829. He retired from the practice of medicine about 1884 at the age of 79 years.

On 7 September 1830, Dr. Chatard married Eliza Ann Marean who was born 13 January 1808 in Martinique, French West Indies. They were married in the Baltimore Basilica. Eight children were born to this couple as listed below. One of his daughters, Juliana Marean Chatard became a religious at St. Joseph's Novitiate in Emmittsburg where she was the mother of novices. A son, Silas Francis Marean Chatard was a Catholic priest, at one time head of the American College in Rome and last serving as the Bishop of Vincennes in Indiana.

Dr. Chatard died on 18 October 1888. The *Baltimore News American* described his demise as follows:

> Dr. Ferdinand Edme Chatard, the venerable and eminent physician of this city, died

Alternative Genealogical Source 1829-1883

suddenly yesterday afternoon of apoplexy at a quarter past four o'clock at his home, No. 516 Park Avenue. He had been in his usual good health during the day, having been out in the morning and again in the afternoon as late as half past two o'clock. He had taken ill while in his bath, about four o'clock and although attended with great skill and care, died about fifteen minutes afterward.

Further, he was described as "being extremely modest and retiring, though deeply and sincerely beloved by neighbors, patients and friends. His associates were almost entirely men in his own profession and among them were such eminent physicians as the late Prof. Nathan R. Smith, Drs. Stewart, McKenzie and Buckler – all his contemporaries. He would never accept any of the many professorships tendered him. During his career he went through the two epidemics of cholera and the many outbreaks of yellow and other fevers."

Dr. Chatard, his parents, children and many other relatives are buried in New Cathedral Cemetery.

Children of Ferdinand Edme and Eliza Ann Marean Chatard are as follows:

1. Julianna Marean Chatard 27 January 1833 – 26 April 1917
2. Silas Francis Marean Chatard 13 December 1834-7 September 1918
3. Francis Peter Chatard 29 October 1836-3 August 1859. A physician who was accidentally drowned at age 22 in Baltimore's harbor.

4. Ferdinand Edme Chatard, Jr. 7 October 1839-27 August 1900. He earned his M.D. from the University of Maryland in 1861. He married Josephine Miles.
5. Mary Tiffany Chatard 31 July 1841-11 January 1870
6. Elizabeth Ann Chatard 31 August 1843-10 February 1847
7. Josephine Mary Chatard 21 May 1845-20 January 1878. She married Philip von Phul in 1870.
8. Thomas Marean Chatard 15 December 1848-15 December 1927. He married Eleanor A. Williams.

The Obstetrical Records

Dr. Pierre Chatard's journals include two large volumes beginning in 1829 and ending in 1846 just prior to his death. These registers are handwritten in French and are very tedious to read. These volumes have not been transcribed here because of the difficulty in reading the entries. Although the handwriting is difficult, at least the names of the women are relatively easy to scan. He begins each new entry with "Mad." in large letters followed by the surname. Mad. is short for Madame or Mrs. in English. Interestingly, most of the surnames are British or Irish. Among those I recognized are the following: Clarke, Richardson, Hawkins, Kirk, Thornton, Hartzell, Miller, Robinson and Kennedy.

Dr. Ferdinand Edme Chatard begins his obstetrical journal in 1829. There are three volumes, the first covers 1829 through 1831. It is small and reveals an evolving style as well as practice. The early entries do not include a full date, but all entries provide exquisite detail of the medical aspects of each case, some covering four, five and six pages for a day-to-day narrative.

The second volume, which is a large register is physically the best preserved. It covers years 1837 through 1850. The medical details decrease, as the number of deliveries increase. Also he begins to formalize his style, so that each entry is more or less similar. His practice is also evolving as he sees more women from prominent Baltimore families and fewer entries for slaves and orphans from St. Vincent's Asylum.

Volume three covers the years 1851 through 1884. This register is in the poorest physical state, the binding having completely broken away. The style of the entries is much the same including date, woman's name, number of previous pregnancies, course of the woman's confinement, gender of the child and details of any complications. In this volume he changes (roughly in 1863) from describing the birth number of the child to the number of the woman's pregnancy. This is of course pertinent when there are multiple births (twins, triplets). This final volume also demonstrates the evolution of Dr. Chatard's practice. As the number of his patient's increase, he takes more time away from the practice, usually in the month of August. It also details the decline in his practice as he ages and slows down.

All of Dr. Ferdinand Edme Chatard's obstetrical registers are written in English. His handwriting is easier to read than that of his father but he has some unique characters that require a little practice to discern. In particular, he seldom closes the *o's* in his words which sometimes makes interpretation of surnames difficult. He also uses a very unusual scripted number *3* which is easily confused with the number *5*. Interpretation of his handwriting is probably the greatest source of error in these transcriptions. Of course, there is some variability in Dr. Chatard's spelling as well. For example, Stuart and Stewart are probably the same surname. McNamara is spelled Mcnemare and sometimes his French ethnicity sneaks in as well such as when Orville becomes Orvaulx. The surname Rennick is probably the same as Renwick and Danman and Damman are likely the same family. There are many more such examples that the user of this index will need to consider.

The transcriptions made here are not full copies of the original entries but rather serve as an index to surnames, dates, child's gender and comments. To provide a better flavor of his work, the following entries were transcribed in their entirety. They are interesting because of the detail concerning the women, the medical treatments and the style of writing. Much of this is a bit foreign to modern medical practice.

Please note, that these entries describe many medical aspects of birth. There is a lot of medical jargon as well as what some may consider gory details. For an explanation of some of the medical terms, see below under *Terminology*.

Alternative Genealogical Source 1829-1883

An early example from volume I, his 26th recorded case:

> *21 August 1830. #26. Mrs. Quinn in labor with fourth child. Called to see her at 2 o'clock AM. She said she had been suffering during the last twelve hours but that the pains had become less a little before I arrived. They were then very slight & returning but every fifteen or twenty minutes. I examined but the os uteri was beyond my reach. I examined again about 5 o'clock. The pains having continued much the same even less. I found the os uteri dilated about the size of a quarter of a dollar. The pains continued rather though not much stronger until about 9 o'clock. The os uteri dilated considerably the waters forming a large & distended pouch. The head of the child appearing to rest on the symphysis of pubis & neither advancing nor receding, it appeared not to touch the os uteri. This continued until about half past eleven & finding the pains considerable the dilatation sufficient for passage child's head & the head not making any advance & moreover suspecting that it rested on the symphysis & the promontory of sacrum, I ruptured the membranes and ... to give a more oblique direction to the head of child. It appeared to me that all my attempts made little or no change in the extraction of the head. A great deal of water escaped & the pains increased greatly after rupture of membranes. At a quarter past one PM, the head had scarce made any progress*

although the pains had been very violent & yet they appeared to me not affect much the head of child. On examining about ten minutes after during a violent pain, I found unexpectedly that the head had greatly advanced & was almost pressing on raphe; in about fifteen or twenty minutes after the child expelled. It was a boy & weighed rather more than nine pounds. The placenta was extracted about half an hour after birth of child having been slight adherent.

An entry from the early portion of his second register describing a miscarriage at eight weeks:

3 October 1837. #262. Mrs. Washington March abortus of about eight weeks was called to her on September 27th. Was informed that she was troubled with a light discharge for several days. Prescribed rest and cold lemonade. By then the discharge was somewhat diminished but it returned toward night with more violence and a good many coagula were passed ... returned again on night of 30th. Several doses of ergot were given by the nurse; they produced great sickness and vomiting. The discharge however cleared almost entirely. ... she was pretty comfortable during the day and the following, having but little pain and less discharge. A dose of Castor oil was given on the 5th which operated very well. On the evening of the third I examined and found ... sufficiently dilated and extracted the after birth which adhered considerably.

Alternative Genealogical Source 1829-1883

Dr. Chatard delivered all of his own children and recorded the details of the births in his journals. Here is the description of the delivery of his son Ferdinand Edme Chatard, Jr., who also became a physician in Baltimore:

> *7 October 1839. #422. Mrs. C* [in another hand F. E. Chatard] *in labor of fourth child had slight pains through the day of 6th about 10 PM the pains became stronger. Os twice dilated about the size of a dollar. Vertex presenting in first position. The labour proceeded regularly and the child was born at a quarter of one a.m. Sex a boy. The placenta was extracted without difficulty. Some difficulty occurred in the passage of the shoulders from the left arm being turned behind the back.*

Here is an example from the height of his career in 1875 that is a long account for that time frame. It describes the birth of twins and post-partum complications leading to the death of the mother:

> *4 July 1875. #4990. Mrs. J. H. Smith 1st pregnancy – called in consultation by Dr. Van Bibber and saw her about 1 PM. I was informed that she was taken in the night and early with a violent convulsion which had been preceded by a very severe headache, after the time I saw her she had had 12 convulsions & had been unconscious since the first. She had been cupped very freely along the spine & ice bags to the head. Hypodermic injections of chloral had been used. On examining I found the os dilated*

about the extent of half a dollar. Vertex presentation in the first portion as she was of full habit. I advised free venisection after bleeding she had but few convulsions but was unconscious & her respiration very labored. Saw her again about 4 PM. Os being somewhat more dilated I ruptured the membranes and as she [cannot read] was difficult we administered ergot hypodermically & gave injections per os of whiskey & assafatidin [?]. Saw her again about 8 PM & the dilatation being sufficient we decided to apply the forceps. The child being removed, we found another presenting one arm & the side of head. I pushed back the arm & altered the position of head so as to apply the forceps. The children were both girls & gave no evidence of life. The placenta which was double was somewhat adherent & required the introduction of the hand to detach it. We gave several doses of Ergot by the mouth. Saw her about 10 AM on 5th. She had pretty fair night, had only one convulsion about 9 AM. Consciousness returned very slowly. At 10 AM on 7th she was decidedly better & in a fair way to recovery. The statement of the attendants that consciousness had returned proved to be erroneous. Although there was some improvement in her case, it did not continue and she died on the 11th July.

As Dr. Chatard's practice grew, his clientele changed. By the mid-point of his practice there are many prominent surnames from Baltimore's society including Carroll, Dulaney, Bonaparte, Jenkins,

Alternative Genealogical Source 1829-1883

Latrobe, Abell, Brown, Hopkins, Buchannon, McComas, Towson and many others. Here is a particularly interesting entry in this regard:

> *9 June 1851 #1983. Mrs. Jerome N. Bonaparte in labour of 2nd child, her first child was born in 1830 about one year after her marriage & she has never been pregnant since, consequently nearly 21 years have elapsed between the two births. Called to her about half past six A.M. Pains regular & strong os quite dilated & she had descended & pressing on vulva, position first of vertex. The child was born about 7 A.M. sex a boy. The placenta was removed without difficulty.*

All levels of Baltimore's society can be found in these journals. Of particular interest to the Afro-American researcher, Dr. Chatard makes note of slaves and "colored" women belonging to their white masters. Here are two such entries:

> *27 June 1843 #862. Dianah a colored woman belonging to Mrs. Henry Mitchell in labour of first child. Called to her about ½ past 11 P.M. Pains strong & frequent. Os nearly entirely dilated, vertex presenting in the first position. Labour natural. The child was born a little before 1 o'clock A.M. Sex a girl. The placenta was removed without difficulty.*

> *7 May 1846 #1279. Rebecca a colored woman belonging to Mr. C. R. Carroll attended by a midwife. She was delivered of*

a first child & the placenta not being expelled one hour & a half after ... it was extracted without difficulty. This patient has a number of small tumors attached to the womb.

Free black women are also included among Dr. Chatard's clientele. The following entry does not note her status, although there are other entries that report her as a married "colored" woman and no notation is ever made of her "belonging" to a master:

26 May 1843 #106. Mrs. Romeo Price (vide July 2nd 1833) Pregnant of her eleventh child. Was sent for at 5 o'clock a.m. Was informed that she had been suffering for sometime. Just before I arrived the waters broke & were followed by a hemorrhage during which she lost about three pints of blood. On examining I found the vagina filled with clots, removed them, then passing of the finger, discovered the knee presenting. I drew it down & then pulled slightly on it, for the purpose of inciting expulsion efforts on the part of the uterus; pain having ceased entirely. Not succeeding in this I gave ten grains ergot, about 15 minutes after the pains came on & the child was expelled. It was about six months old & dead. The placenta was extracted without difficulty. No further hemorrhage occurred. The mother did well.

Alternative Genealogical Source 1829-1883

Statistics

The following charts and reports manipulate the data extracted from the registers of Dr. Chatard's journals to reflect his practice and the patient's within that practice.

The following graph demonstrates the growth, stability and demise of Dr. Chatard's obstetrical practice from 1829 when he delivered six patients to 1857, the zenith of his annual deliveries at 178 and finally to 1883 when at age 78 he delivered five women. His numbers peak just before the Civil War. The subsequent decline may reflect his advancing age but probably in part also reflects the national economic troubles of 1857/1858, the loss of young men during the war and the increasing competition as more and more medical schools in the city graduated new physicians.

Obstetrical Casebooks of Dr. F. E. Chatard

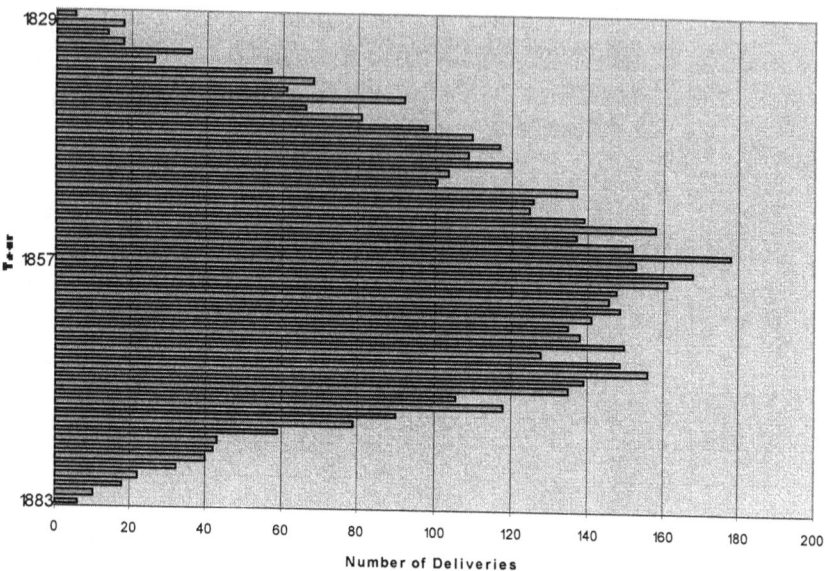

Dr. Ferdinand E. Chatard Deliveries 1829-1883

Of the 5,285 deliveries in Dr. Chatard's three volumes, the gender of the child is provided in 5,140 deliveries or 5,281 children when multiple births are counted. Males account for 50.6% and females 49.4%. There are 54 twin births. Of these 23 were twin girls, 16 twin boys and 15 one of each (of the latter interestingly, 12 were male/female births while only three were female/male births). There was one set of triplets born prematurely at six months. They did not survive. The triplets consisted of two males and one female.

The peak number of pregnancies for women in Dr. Chatard's practice was five. Of those having ten or more pregnancies, the numbers break down as follows:

Alternative Genealogical Source 1829-1883

10	11	12	13	14	15	16	17
63	49	26	23	8	3	3	1

Table 1. Women with 10 or more pregnancies

Mrs. James Dougherty gave birth to her 17th child on Independence Day 1821!

Births recorded at St. Vincent's Asylum (an orphanage) numbered 54.

Births for "colored" women numbered about 100.

Dr. Chatard delivered the following number of children on holidays:

25 December (Christmas)	15
1 January (New Years)	16
4 July (Independence Day)	14
5 August (his birthday)	21
13 January (his wife's birthday)	19
7 September (his wedding anniversary)	19

Table 2. Dr. Chatard worked on these holidays

Notes on Content and Organization

The main body of this work is an index to volumes I through III of Dr. Ferdinand Edme Chatard's obstetrical journals which cover fifty-five years of deliveries in Baltimore City from 1829 until 1883. In total there are 5,285 deliveries described, although Dr. Chatard's original entries are numbered through 5,265. The difference of twenty entries is because on rare occasion he failed to number all of the entries and at least once, he made a mistake in the numbering system.

The entries are arranged alphabetically by surname. The woman's first name is given in the second column. Unfortunately, especially in the early years this is often just "Mrs." and sometimes is completely blank. The latter is most often found for entries of slaves, unmarried mothers and inmates of St. Vincent's Asylum.

The third column is the date of the child's birth. The fourth column is Dr. Chatard's numbered entry. This is provided because it will make it very easy to locate the original entry. As always in transcription projects of this nature, if you locate an entry of interest in this index, I encourage you to check the original in the Special Collections division of the Furlong Baldwin Library of the Maryland Historical Society in Baltimore City.

The fifth column is the child's gender, M for male, F for female. Occasionally, Dr. Chatard forgets to enter the child's sex. This will occur most often when there is a miscarriage, which is likely an intentional omission, but also sometimes with routine deliveries he neglects to include the child's gender.

Alternative Genealogical Source 1829-1883

The sixth and last column records pertinent details from the birth entry. Almost always, Dr. Chatard recorded either the number of the child (in birth sequence) or the number of the pregnancy. Sometimes, he obviously doesn't know and the space has been left blank. Sometimes, when you follow an individual woman sequentially through these registers the numbers are not consistent. In part this may be because he sometimes refers to the number of the child (first, second third, etc. child) and sometimes he refers to the number of the pregnancy. These are not always the same value when one includes miscarriages and multiple births.

Also in this last column, I occasionally directly quote from the original record some interesting or unique fact such as circumstances describing when the mother or child dies or if a birth was complicated.

Terminology

Not surprisingly, there is a lot of medical jargon in Dr. Chatard's obstetrical registers. In my index, I avoided as much of this as possible, however if the reader uses the original work, the following may be of some assistance. Some of these are easily recognized medical terms, mostly anatomical. A lot of his descriptive terms are peculiar to the nineteenth-century. This is not an all-inclusive list.

Abortion: as used here, Dr. Chatard means a spontaneous miscarriage, not intentional termination of a pregnancy. Sometimes he uses the Latin *abortus* to refer to the fetus.

Obstetrical Casebooks of Dr. F. E. Chatard

Antimony: had many indications including expectorant, diaphoretic and emetic. This agent is no longer used in modern medical care.

Attended by: most often he uses this phrase when his medical skills have been requested by another physician, midwife or sometimes even the patient. Occasionally, he will actually state that he was asked to see the patient in consultation, but most often he will simply state that the patient was attended by Dr. So-and-So. Quite frequently, Dr. VanBibber is the attending physician. He was related to Dr. Chatard by marriage.

Bismuth: this agent was used as a cathartic. Depending on the salt, this agent could be used for a variety of other indications including treatment of wounds and ulcers and various infections.

Bleeding: a technique whereby the skin was lanced to allow deliberate blood loss. Different sized lancets would produce unique lacerations and provide treatment for a variety of medical problems. The pulse (both rate and quality) was measured to determine whether an appropriate response had been attained. Bleeding was indicated for many conditions including ironically hemorrhage. This 19th-century technique persisted well into the early decades of the 20th-century but is no longer part of modern medical care.

Breech: feet or bottom first delivery

Chloroform: an early means of anesthesia introduced in 1847. Although Dr. Chatard mentions this frequently (sometimes as *chloral* which is probably not a reference to chloral hydrate but rather abbreviation for chloroform) as a "state of the art" medication in his practice, it has long ago been replaced by other means, most often now epidural anesthesia. Chloroform was made known round the world when administered to Queen Victoria during pregnancy. It is potentially lethal and can actually retard delivery.

Coagula: In Dr. Chatard's notes this refers to blood clots often associated with hemorrhage.

Confinement: defines the experience of childbirth or more specifically the time that the woman was in labor and post-partum recovery. Dr. Chatard most frequently uses this terminology when he describes a woman's death. For example, she died in the fifth day of her confinement means that she died five days after the birth of her child.

Convulsion: this term is a nineteenth-century description of a seizure. Seizures occur during pregnancy most often during what is now labeled eclampsia. This is a condition characterized by fluid retention, hypertension and increased risk to the mother and child. Many of Dr. Chatard's descriptions of convulsions also note edema (fluid retention), anasarca (massive fluid retention) and changes in mental status such as unconsciousness.

Cupping: not a procedure unique to obstetrics. Cupping was accomplished by heating a small glass bell and applying it to the skin, essentially creating a hot vacuum which in turned caused the skin to redden and blister. This is not a part of modern medical care.

Ergot: or ergotamines are derived from a fungus infecting rye. Ergot has been used to induce uterine contractions and peripheral blood vasoconstriction. Dr. Chatard uses this agent frequently in slow labor or especially when there is hemorrhage.

Forceps: an instrument used to grasp and pull or turn a child during birth providing traction. There are a variety of forceps designed to accomplish different tasks. Dr. Chatard gives names to different instruments in his collection. He often notes that he sent someone to bring his forceps from his home.

Laudanum: a 19th-century term for opium or more specifically a tincture of opium.

Opium: derived from the poppy plant and administered as an analgesic. Used not infrequently during the 19th-century. Today morphine and other narcotic agents are employed.

Os uterus: the opening or literally the mouth of the uterus through which the child must pass. Dr. Chatard uniformly describes the size by comparison to quarters, half-dollars and dollar coins. Today the standard terminology is to estimate the diameter in centimeters and to report it as so-many centimeters of dilatation.

Placenta: medical term for lay-term "afterbirth"

Position: Dr. Chatard always describes the child's position within the womb as *first position, second position* or *third position*. These now archaic terms define the progress of delivery as well as the alignment of the child in the mother's womb.

Symphysis: midline of the boney pelvis over which the child passes during birth.

Vertex: head first delivery

Venisection: the same as bleeding.

References

Baltimore American, "End of life of a beloved physician – his many noble qualities." 19 October 1888, p. 4, col.B.

Haubrich MD, William S. *Medical Meanings, a Glossary of Word Origins.* Harcourt Brace Jovanovich Publishers, 1984.

Medical and Chirurgical Faculty of Maryland Manuscript Collection, 1773-1975. MS 3000. Maryland Historical Society Special Collections. Box labeled Chatard. Folder: Chatard, Ferdinand Edme, Obstetrical Case Records 1829-37 C/MSS/27976.

Medical and Chirurgical Faculty of Maryland Manuscript Collection, 1773-1975. MS 3000. Maryland Historical Society Special Collections. Box labeled Chatard. Folders: (1) Chatard,

Obstetrical Casebooks of Dr. F. E. Chatard

Ferdinand Edme, Obstetrical Case Records 1837-1850 and (2) Chatard, Ferdinand Edme, Obstetrical Case Records 1851-1883.

Medical and Chirurgical Faculty of Maryland Manuscript Collection, 1773-1975. MS 3000. Maryland Historical Society Special Collections. Box labeled Chatard. Folders: (1) Chatard, Pierre, Obstetrical Case Records 1828-1835 and (2) Chatard, Pierre, Obstetrical Case Records 1836-1846.

Merck's 1899 Manual of the Materia Medica. NewYork: Merck & Co., 1899.

Sexton Records, New Cathedral Cemetery. Chatard Family Plot, Section KK, lots 96 through 99.

Taylor MD, E. Stewart. *Obstetrics.* Baltimore: Williams & Wilkins Company, 1972.

Williams MD, Leonard. *Minor Maladies and their treatment.* Baltimore: William Wood and Company, 1934.

Young, Dixie Walker, (compiler) *The Chatard Family Journal*: Volume number I, January 1978 – Volume number 11, 1982. Idaho Falls, Idaho: Chatard Family Organization, 1978-1982. Maryland Historical Society Library call number CS71.C492.

Obstetrical Casebooks of Dr. F. E. Chatard – an alternative genealogical resource 1829-1883

Surname	Given Name	No.	Date	Sex	Comments
[--?--]	[--?--]	20	13-Dec-1830		colored at Center St., first child
[--?--]	[--?--]	59	09-Dec-1832	M	a colored woman belonging to Mrs. Leach, sixth child
[--?--]	[--?--]	74	05-May-1833	F	colored woman at Centre St attended by Dr. Gratham. "My father and myself saw her." Child dead
[--?--]	[--?--]	75	06-May-1833	M	colored woman, a slave of Mr. Waring on Courtland St., third child, child dead
[--?--]	[--?--]	91	After 26 Nov, before 23 Dec 1833		a servant of Mrs. Ringold. Attended by midwife.
[--?--]	[--?--]	189	24-May-1836		a servant of Mrs. Siday Winder, retained placenta
[--?--]	[--?--]	208	27-Sep-1836	M	a colored woman of W. Tiffany, second child
[--?--]	[--?--]	267	06-Nov-1837	F	a colored woman belonging to Mrs. Lafone
[--?--]	[--?--]	1033	01-Sep-1844	M	colored woman belonging to Mrs. Austin Jenkins, 3rd child
[--?--]	Adeline	3344	25-Feb-1860	M	colored servant of Mrs. A. Harris, 14 years old
[--?--]	Agnes	2810	19-Oct-1856	M	colored, second child
[--?--]	Agnes	2966	18-Sep-1857	F	at St. Vincent's Asylum
[--?--]	Agnes	3105	28-Jul-1858	M	at St. Vincent's Asylum, first child
[--?--]	Amelia	3575	29-Sep-1861	F	at St. Vincent's Insane Asylum, first child
[--?--]	Amey	97	22-Feb-1834	F	colored woman, second child
[--?--]	Ann	3937	16-Oct-1864	M	at St. Vincent's Asylum, first pregnancy, premature "It lived but two days."
[--?--]	Anney	3201	25-Feb-1859	F/F	a colored woman of Mrs. Mary Brown, five month pregnancy, twins
[--?--]	Annie	3019	18-Dec-1857	F	at St. Vincent's Asylum
[--?--]	Annie	3407	19-Aug-1860	M	St. Vincent's Asylum, 1st child

1

Obstetrical Casebooks of Dr. F. E. Chatard – an alternative genealogical resource 1829-1883

[-?-]	Annie	4451	17-May-1869	F	second pregnancy
[-?-]	Augusta	4262	13-Oct-1867	F	at St. Vincent's Asylum
[-?-]	Augusta	4341	14-Jun-1868	F	at St. Vincent's Insane Asylum, first pregnancy
[-?-]	Betsy	219	10-Jan-1837	M	colored woman belonging to Mrs. W. Tiffany
[-?-]	Bridget	3509	17-Apr-1861	M	at St. Vincent's Asylum, first child
[-?-]	Catherine	3040	03-Feb-1858	F	at St. Vincent's Asylum, first child
[-?-]	Charlotte	66	29-Jan-1833	M	colored, second child, child dead
[-?-]	Dinah	862	27-Jun-1843	F	colored be-longing to Mrs. Hnry Mitchell, 1st child
[-?-]	Elisabeth	3273	15-Sep-1859	F	St. Vincent's Asylum, 2nd child
[-?-]	Eliza	1208	25-Sep-1845	M	a bound woman attended by a midwife
[-?-]	Emily	500	15-Jun-1840	M	a colored woman at Mrs. Treadwells, first
[-?-]	Eveline	3221	17-Apr-1859	M	at St. Vincent's Asylum, first child
[-?-]	Florence	3189	22-Jan-1859	M	at St. Vincent's Asylum, first child
[-?-]	Frances	3520	11-May-1861	M	colored woman belonging to A. Schaffer
[-?-]	Francisqua	24	28-Jun-1831	M	a servant of Mrs. Dalla Costa & an Indian from the banks of the Bonokie, second child
[-?-]	Harriette	2905	24-May-1857	F	first child
[-?-]	Josephine	2856	27-Jan-1857	M	first child, St. Vincent's Asylum
[-?-]	Josephine	3825	27-Nov-1863	M	at St. Vincent's Asylum, first pregnancy
[-?-]	Julia	3403	02-Aug-1860	F	at St. Vincent's Asylum, first child
[-?-]	Julia	3740	24-Jan-1863	F	at St. Vincent's Asylum, first child
[-?-]	Julia	3778	23-May-1863	M	at St. Vincent's Asylum, first child
[-?-]	Julia	3813	26-Sep-1863	M	at St. Vincent's Asylum
[-?-]	Kesiah	1146	10-May-1845		colored woman belonging to Mrs. J. Bowdoin, first child, died after a few hours
[-?-]	Lorett	3518	07-May-1861	F	at St. Vincent's Asylum, first child

2

Obstetrical Casebooks of Dr. F. E. Chatard – an alternative genealogical resource 1829-1883

[-?-]	Lucy	1608	02-Aug-1848	M	colored woman belonging to Mrs. J. Nonges
[-?-]	Lucy	2831	27-Nov-1856	M	at St. Vincent's Asylum, first child
[-?-]	Lydia	3101	24-Jul-1858	F	first child
[-?-]	Madeleine	673	17-Jan-1842	M	colored, first child
[-?-]	Madeleine	2858	04-Feb-1857	M	first child, St. Mary's Asylum
[-?-]	Margaret	2893	22-Apr-1857	F	first child, at St. Vincent's Asylum
[-?-]	Margaret	3257	21-Jul-1859	F	at St. Vincent's Asylum, first child
[-?-]	Margaret	4554	26-May-1870	M	at St. Vincent's Asylum, attended by Drs. VanBibber & Brewer, child dead
[-?-]	Maria	64	26-Jan-1833	F	colored, fourth child, child appeared dead but was "restored."
[-?-]	Maria	3001	14-Nov-1857	M	at St. Vincent's Asylum, first child
[-?-]	Maria	3379	06-Jun-1860	F	at St. Vincent's Asylum, first child
[-?-]	Mary	4			residing in Waggon Alley, first child; "It did not readily suck."
[-?-]	Mary	6		M	colored, aged 16, first child; child died
[-?-]	Mary	473	26-Mar-1840	F	a colored woman belonging to Mrs. Caton
[-?-]	Mary	736	16-Jul-1842	F	colored, first child
[-?-]	Mary	3060	22-Mar-1858	M	at St. Vincent's Asylum, first child
[-?-]	Mary	3190	23-Jan-1859	M	at St. Vincent's Asylum, first child
[-?-]	Mary	3264	23-Aug-1859		at St. Vincent's Asylum, first child
[-?-]	Mary	5013	21-Oct-1875	M	first pregnancy, illegitimate
[-?-]	Mary Augusta	3697	01-Nov-1862	F	at St. Vincent's Asylum, first child
[-?-]	Mary Elizabeth	4028	09-Sep-1865		at St. Vincent's Orphan Asylum), first pregnancy
[-?-]	Matilda	3093	06-Jun-1858	M/M	at St. Vincent's Asylum, twins
[-?-]	Miss	196	01-Aug-1836	M	second child, child dead

Obstetrical Casebooks of Dr. F. E. Chatard – an alternative genealogical resource 1829-1883

[--?--]	Miss	365	14-Feb-1839	F	miscarriage at four months
[--?--]	Miss	472	26-Mar-1840		first child
[--?--]	Miss	961	12-Feb-1844	M	first child
[--?--]	Miss	1655	22-Dec-1848	F	first pregnancy, 5.5 months, fetus dead
[--?--]	Miss	5061	24-Jun-1876	F	first child
[--?--]	Miss Annie	3413	03-Sep-1860		at St. Vincent's Asylum, first child
[--?--]	Miss Elisabeth	3411	30-Aug-1860	M	at St. Vincent's Asylum, first child
[--?--]	Miss Laura	3501	15-Mar-1861	F	at St. Vincent's Asylum, first pregnancy
[--?--]	Miss Lizzie	3969	05-Jan-1865	F	St. Vincent's Asylum, forceps delivery. "There was a feeble pulsation of the heart when born but soon ceased."
[--?--]	Miss Louisa	3935	09-Oct-1864	M	first child. "I used chloroform in this case with advantage."
[--?--]	Miss Margaret	2421	10-May-1854	F	first child
[--?--]	Miss Matilde	2873	05-Mar-1857	M	first child, in fifth month
[--?--]	Mrs.	973	24-Mar-1844	F	at St. Vincent's Asylum, third child. "Attended during my absence by my son."
[--?--]	Mrs.	3463	12-Dec-1860	M	first pregnancy
[--?--]	Mrs. Kate	4759	10-Jun-1872	M	colored at home of Thomas Alexander, first child
[--?--]	Nellie	2668	11-Oct-1855	M	colored woman at J. Campbell White
[--?--]	Phoebe	1291	16-Jun-1846	M	a colored woman at Mrs. J. Buchannans, 3rd
[--?--]	Rachel	470	20-Mar-1840	F	colored woman belonging to Mrs. C. R. Carroll, first child
[--?--]	Rebecca	1279	07-May-1846		at St. Vincent's Asylum, first pregnancy
[--?--]	Rosalie	3807	20-Aug-1863	F	at St. Vincent's Asylum, first child
[--?--]	Rose	3151	21-Oct-1858	M	colored
[--?--]	Rosine	859	21-Jun-1843	M	at St. Vincent's Asylum, first child
[--?--]	Sally	2834	30-Nov-1856	M	

4

Obstetrical Casebooks of Dr. F. E. Chatard – an alternative genealogical resource 1829-1883

[--?--]	Sophia	1712	02-Jun-1849	M/F	colored woman belonging to Mrs. Biscoe, twins, daughter dead
[--?--]	Sophia	3839	12-Jan-1865	M	at St. Vincent's Asylum, first pregnancy
[--?--]	Stella	3016	09-Dec-1857	F	at St. Vincent's Asylum
[--?--]	Susan	2985	21-Oct-1857	F/F	at St. Vincent's Asylum, second child, twins, stillborn
[--?--]	Susan	3070	11-Apr-1858	M	at St. Vincent's Asylum, first child, forceps
Abell	Mrs. G. W.	4918	04-Aug-1874	F	second pregnancy
Abell	Mrs. George W.	4791	31-Oct-1872	F	first pregnancy
Abell	Mrs. George W.	5062	25-Jun-1875	M	third pregnancy
Abercrombie	Mrs. John	4120	20-Jul-1866	F	first pregnancy
Abercrombie	Mrs. John	4223	06-Jun-1867	M	second pregnancy
Abrahams	Mrs. H. W. D.	5256	21-Jul-1882	F	third pregnancy, "Being obliged to change her residence, she rode about half a mile. During the ride the membranes gave way …."
Acton	Mrs. S. G.	2471	29-Aug-54	M	first child
Adair	Mrs.	341	12-Oct-1838	M	third child
Adair	Mrs. T.	445	29-Dec-1839	M	fourth child
Adams	Mrs. Capt. G.	2082	14-Jan-1852	F	attended by Dr. Rider
Adams	Mrs. Edward	2827	18-Nov-1856	M	first child. "Gave no sign of life."
Adams	Mrs. J. M.	4182	27-Jan-1867	F	third pregnancy
Adams	Mrs. J. M.	4385	12-Nov-1868	M	fourth pregnancy
Adams	Mrs. Joseph	3542	12-Jul-1861	M	fifth pregnancy
Adams	Mrs. Joseph	3841	13-Jan-1864	M	sixth pregnancy
Adams	Mrs. Joseph S.	3280	10-Oct-1859	M	fourth child
Addison	Mrs. W. M.	1658	02-Jan-1849	M	second child
Addison	Mrs. Wm. M.	1439	26-May-1847	M	first child
Addison	Mrs. Wm. M.	4122	25-Jul-1866	F	third pregnancy
Addison	Mrs. Wm. Mead	2880	15-Mar-1857	F	fifth child

Obstetrical Casebooks of Dr. F. E. Chatard – an alternative genealogical resource 1829-1883

Addison	Mrs. Wm. Mead	3865	13-Mar-1864	F	second pregnancy
Addison	Mrs. Wm. Meade	2539	15-Jan-1855	M	fourth child
Ahern	Mrs.	244	19-Aug-1837	M	first child
Ahern	Mrs.	332	12-Sep-1838	F	second child
Ahern	Mrs. M.	547	24-Nov-1840	F	third child
Ahern	Mrs. T. J.	779	17-Nov-1842	F	fourth child
Aigerberger	Mrs. Phillip	3538	02-Jul-1861	M	third child
Aikin	Mrs.	838	18-Apr-1843	F	sixth child
Aikin	Mrs. Dr.	1411	28-Mar-1847	M	born 10 AM
Aikin	Mrs. Dr.	1979	25-May-1851	M	fourth child
Aikin	Mrs. Dr. R.	2286	27-May-1853	M	seventh child
Aikin	Mrs. Dr. R. E.	1693	20-Mar-1849	M	fourth child
Aikin	Mrs. Dr. Wm.	2959	06-Sep-1857	M	sixth child, attended by Dr Chew
Aikins	Mrs. Professor	2452	25-Jul-1854	M	fourth child
Aker	Mrs.	425	15-Oct-1839		miscarriage at 3 months
Aker	Mrs. Michael	359	11-Jan-1839	F	second child
Aker	Mrs. Michael	653	03-Nov-1841	M	third child
Aker	Mrs. Michael	847	15-May-1843	F	fourth child
Aker	Mrs. Michael	1135	08-Mar-1845	M	large male child
Albert	Mrs. Augustus	2622	19-Jul-1855	M	first child
Albert	Mrs. J.	1752	23-Sep-1849	M	born 5 AM
Albert	Mrs. W.	3495	25-Feb-1861	M	11th child
Albert	Mrs. Wm. J.	1931	29-Dec-1850	M	seventh child
Albert	Mrs. Wm. J.	2638	17-Aug-1855	M	ninth child

Obstetrical Casebooks of Dr. F. E. Chatard – an alternative genealogical resource 1829-1883

Albert	Mrs. Wm. L.	2431	29-May-1854	M	eighth child
Albert	Mrs. Wm. T.	2991	29-Oct-1857	M	tenth child
Aler	Mrs. J.	1017	28-Jul-1844	M	third child
Aler	Mrs. John	1538	01-Feb-1848	M/F	fifth child, twins, girl did not survive
Aler	Mrs. John	2410	12-Apr-1854	M	sixth child
Alexander	Mrs. J. H.	559	14-Dec-1840	F	fourth child. Very difficult delivery. In coma. Delivered three more children. Died at age 79 on 16 Feb 1887
Alexander	Mrs. J. H.	1261	16-Feb-1846	F	see December 14, 1840. Fifth child
Alexander	Mrs. J. H.	1453	12-Jul-1847	M	sixth child
Alexander	Mrs. J. H.	1705	06-May-1849	M	seventh child, mother suffered convulsions
Alexander	Mrs. John H.	1990	19-Jun-1851	M	eighth child
Alexander	Mrs. Thomas	1225	06-Nov-1845	F	ninth child
Allan	Mrs. John	3528	29-May-1861	M	first child
Allen	Mrs. H.	2028	28-Sep-1851	F	seventh child
Allen	Mrs. Henry	2397	24-Feb-1854	M	eighth child
Allen	Mrs. Henry	2687	03-Dec-1855	F	ninth child
Allen	Mrs. Henry	3099	19-Jul-1858	M	born about 10 AM
Allen	Mrs. Henry	3499	13-Mar-1861	M	11th child
Allen	Mrs. Louis	4125	30-Jul-1866	F	second pregnancy
Allen	Mrs. W.	206	20-Sep-1836	M	second child
Almire	Mrs.	2319	09-Aug-1853	F	second child
Almond	Margaret	2354	13-Nov-1853	F	colored, first child
Alrick	Mrs. F. W.	2043	22-Oct-1851	F	sixth child
Alricks	Mrs. Francis	803	02-Jan-1843	F	second child
Alricks	Mrs. Francis	1095	31-Dec-1844	F	fifth child
Anderson	Mrs. Adner	4022	27-Aug-1855	M	third pregnancy

7

Obstetrical Casebooks of Dr. F. E. Chatard – an alternative genealogical resource 1829-1883

Anderson	Mrs. Adner	4242	15-Aug-1867	M	fourth pregnancy
Anderson	Mrs. Robert S.	3972	14-Jan-1865	M	fourth pregnancy
Anspach	Mrs. F. R.	3599	18-Dec-1861	F	second child
Appleton	Mrs. W. S.	2301	04-Jul-1853	F	ninth child
Arango	Mrs.	15	29-Jun-1830	M	35-years old, first child, child did not live
Ardin	Mrs. D.	585	09-Apr-1841	F	born 12 PM
Ardin	Mrs. D.	3466	17-Dec-1860	F	"… at 12 o'clock at her request I applied the forceps"
Arens	Mrs. H.	2789	02-Sep-1856	F	first child
Armistead	Mrs. C. Hughes	1039	13-Sep-1844	F	second child
Armstrong	Mrs.	112	19-Jul-1834	M	born 10:25 PM
Armstrong	Mrs.	1310	30-Jul-1846		
Armstrong	Mrs. Andrew	605	30-Jun-1841	M	third child
Armstrong	Mrs. Andrew	977	28-Mar-1844	M	third child
Armstrong	Mrs. Hughes	1365	06-Dec-1846	M	first child
Armstrong	Mrs. J. A.	2527	15-Dec-1854	M	sixth child
Armstrong	Mrs. James A.	1581	28-May-1848	F	considerable hemorrhage
Armstrong	Mrs. James A.	1813	13-Feb-1850		third child
Armstrong	Mrs. James A.	2096	05-Feb-1852	F	fourth child
Armstrong	Mrs. James A.	2379	12-Jan-1854	F	fifth child, premature at 7 months, stillborn
Armstrong	Mrs. James D.	1200	04-Sep-1845	F	first child
Arnold	Mrs. G. W.	678	25-Jan-1842	M	born 2 AM
Arthur	Mrs. Charles	3321	10-Jan-1860	M	first child
Arthur	Mrs. Robert	2049	04-Nov-51	M/F	first child, born … very feeble, twins. Both died
Ash	Mrs.	2755	30-May-1856	M	fourth child
Ash	Mrs. L. M.	3219	28-Mar-1859	M	fifth child

8

Obstetrical Casebooks of Dr. F. E. Chatard – an alternative genealogical resource 1829-1883

Ash	Mrs. Louis	3578	20-Oct-1861	M	sixth child
Ash	Mrs. Louis	3903	10-Jul-1864	F	seventh pregnancy
Ash	Mrs. Louis	4107	02-Jun-1866	F	eighth pregnancy
Ash	Mrs. Louis	4621	12-Dec-1870	F	ninth pregnancy
Atkinson	Mrs.	243	04-Aug-1837		first child, still born
Atkinson	Mrs. Dr.	1347	27-Oct-1846	F	second child
Atkinson	Mrs. Dr.	1638	30-Oct-1848	M	third child
Atkinson	Mrs. Dr. T.	1158	22-May-1845	F	first child
Atwell	Mrs.	2158	17-Jul-1852	F	fourth child
Augustus	Mrs. Henry	2461	16-Aug-1854	F	colored, first child
Ault	Mrs. S.	none	07-Aug-1874	F	third pregnancy, attended by Dr. Van Bibber
Ault	Mrs. Samuel	4704	13-Nov-1871	M	second pregnancy
Austin	Mrs.	287	11-Mar-1838	M	
Bachaerache	Mrs. A.	2741	24-Apr-1856	F	Nr. 29 Ensor St. fifth child
Backen	Mrs. A.	3494	19-Feb-1861	F	first child
Baehr	Mrs. Louis	2981	12-Oct-1857	F	fifth child
Baer	Mrs. A. P.	4682	26-Jul-1871	M	second pregnancy
Baer	Mrs. Arthur P.	4991	17-Jul-1875	M	third pregnancy
Baer	Mrs. Arthur P.	4319	29-Mar-1868	F	first pregnancy
Baer	Mrs. Dr. R.	3374	25-May-1860	M	second child
Baer	Mrs. Dr. R.	3656	09-Jul-1862	M	third child
Baer	Mrs. E. R.	3155	01-Nov-1858	F	first child
Baer	Mrs. L.	2274	30-Apr-1853	M	third child
Baer	Mrs. L.	2447	17-Jul-1854	M	fourth child
Bagby	Mrs.	2989	25-Oct-1857	F	second child

Obstetrical Casebooks of Dr. F. E. Chatard – an alternative genealogical resource 1829-1883

Bagby	Mrs. James	3233	14-May-1859	M	third child
Baker	Mrs. W. G.	1224	05-Nov-1845	M	first child. Attacked with puerperal fever and died on the 6th day
Balderstone	Mrs. J. C.	3558	23-Aug-1861	F	first child
Balderstone	Mrs. J. C.	3746	16-Feb-1863	M	second pregnancy
Balderstone	Mrs. J. C.	3987	24-Mar-1865	M	third pregnancy
Balderstone	Mrs. J. C.	4615	04-Dec-1870	M	fifth pregnancy
Balderstone	Mrs. J. C.	4878	17-Jan-1874	M/M	sixth pregnancy, twins, eight months
Balderstone	Mrs. J. C.	4324	14-Apr-1868	M	fourth pregnancy
Balderstone	Mrs. John C.	5083	06-Oct-1876	F	seventh pregnancy
Baldwin	Mrs.	1777	24-Nov-1849	F	third child
Baldwin	Mrs. Charles W.	4495	24-Oct-1869	F	first pregnancy
Baldwin	Mrs. R. T.	1149	14-May-1845	F	first child
Baldwin	Mrs. R. T.	1401	12-Mar-1847	M	second child
Baldwin	Mrs. S.	3497	09-Mar-1861	F	first child
Baldwin	Mrs. S.	3650	25-Jun-1862	M	second child
Baldwin	Mrs. Summerfield	4671	19-Jun-1871	M	first pregnancy
Baldwin	Mrs. Summerfield	4833	12-May-1873	M	second pregnancy
Baldwin	Mrs. Summerfield	4908	14-Jun-1874	F	third pregnancy
Baldwin	Mrs. Summerfield	5070	20-Jul-1876	F	fourth pregnancy
Baldwin	Mrs. W.	4818	25-Feb-1873	F	ninth pregnancy, severe hemorrhage "…applying of ice & vinegar to the womb, Ergot & Brandy as also given."
Baldwin	Mrs. W.H.	4738	08-Mar-1872	M	eighth pregnancy

Obstetrical Casebooks of Dr. F. E. Chatard – an alternative genealogical resource 1829-1883

Baldwin, Jr.	Mrs. W. H.	4602	26-Oct-1870	M	seventh pregnancy
Bandel [?]	Mrs. Dr. W. T.	3272	14-Sep-1859	M	first child
Banks	Mrs. F. F.	988	30-Apr-1844	F	born a little after 4 PM
Banks	Mrs. F. F.	1278	05-May-1846	F	born 11:30 PM
Banks	Mrs. F. F.	1605	27-Jul-1848	F	ninth child
Banks	Mrs. F. F.	1959	05-Mar-1851	M	ninth child
Banks	Mrs. J.	693	12-Mar-1842	F	first child
Banks	Mrs. J. W.	1564	20-Apr-1843	M	born half past twelve midnight
Baqstien	Mrs. Emile	2907	27-May-1857	F	first child
Barclay	Mrs. Grace	2440	19-Jun-1854	M	second child
Barclay	Mrs. Walter	2716	19-Feb-1856	M	third child
Barclay	Mrs. Walter	3010	29-Nov-1857	F	fourth child
Barclay	Mrs. Walter	3309	20-Dec-1859	F	fifth child
Bargan	Mrs. Henry	3064	02-Apr-1858	M	second child
Bargar	Mrs. Henry	2677	08-Nov-1855	M	first child
Bargar	Mrs. Henry	3439	04-Nov-1860	F	third child
Bargar	Mrs. Henry	3699	01-Nov-1862	M	fourth child
Bargar	Mrs. Henry	4141	30-Aug-66		fifth pregnancy
Baris	Mrs. James	4473	05-Aug-69	M	first pregnancy
Barker	Mrs. J. H.	4713	03-Dec-71	M	second pregnancy
Barker	Mrs. Joseph	3744	04-Feb-63	M	first child
Barker	Mrs. Joseph	3968	01-Jan-1865	F	seventh month. "The child lived but a few hours."
Barnard	Mrs. L.	2829	23-Nov-1856	F	second child
Barnes	Mrs.	3261	11-Aug-1859	F	first child, attended by Dr. Chew. "She began to sink soon after and died in about 1/2 an hour."

11

Obstetrical Casebooks of Dr. F. E. Chatard – an alternative genealogical resource 1829-1883

Barnes	Mrs. J. E.	4295	14-Feb-1868	F	sixth pregnancy
Barnes	Mrs. S. E.	3315	31-Dec-1859	F	fourth child
Barnes	Mrs. S. E.	3883	23-Apr-1864	F	sixth pregnancy
Barreda	Mrs. F.	2481	18-Sep-1854	F	first child
Barreeda	Mrs. F.	2723	11-Mar-1856	F	second child
Barrett	Mrs.	685	18-Feb-1842	M	third child
Barrett	Mrs.	1294	20-Jun-1846	F	eighth child
Barrett	Mrs. J.	4925	19-Aug-74	M	sixth pregnancy
Barrett	Mrs. J. J.	4010	30-May-1865	M	second pregnancy
Barrett	Mrs. J. J.	4532	11-Mar-1870	M	the child being born before I arrived
Barrett	Mrs. James	4224	09-Jun-1867	F	third pregnancy
Barrett	Mrs. James J.	3870	24-Mar-1864	F	first pregnancy
Barrett	Mrs. M.	2724	12-Mar-1856		fifth child, dead. " … this being the third occurrence of this kind."
Barringer	Mrs. Marean	2576	27-Mar-1855	F	fourth child
Barringer	Mrs. Thoreau	1701	09-Apr-1849	F	first child
Barroll	Mrs. J. W.	792	15-Dec-1842		first child
Barroll	Mrs. James	1023	14-Aug-44	F	second child
Barroll	Mrs. James	1729	22-Jul-1849	M	fifth child
Barroll	Mrs. James	2948	18-Aug-1857	F	first child
Barroll	Mrs. James	3381	11-Jun-1860	M	second child
Barrow	Mrs. Fk. N.	3964	29-Dec-1864	M	first pregnancy
Barry	Mrs. George E.	2434	02-Jun-1854		first child
Barry	Mrs. J. C.	342	13-Oct-1838	M	born 3 AM
Barry	Mrs. J. S.	3979	31-Jan-1865	M	ninth pregnancy
Barry	Mrs. Llewellyn	3401	02-Aug-1860	M	first child

Obstetrical Casebooks of Dr. F. E. Chatard – an alternative genealogical resource 1829-1883

Barthy	Mrs. P.	2495	09-Oct-1854	F	first child
Bartol	Mrs. J. B.	695	20-Mar-1842	M	fourth child, died at five hours
Bartol	Mrs. N.	168	30-Nov-1835	F	second child
Barton	Mrs.	681	02-Feb-1842	M	first child
Barton	Mrs. D.	5199	15-Aug-1879	M	second pregnancy
Basil	Mrs. John	3754	04-Mar-1863	F	first pregnancy
Basker	Fanney	217	15-Dec-1836		colored, second child, "twelve years having elapsed between the two." unmarried, child dead
Bastien	Mrs. Emile	3505	09-Apr-1865	M	second child
Bastien	Mrs. Emile	4102	11-May-1866	M	third pregnancy
Batten	Mrs.	2296	18-Jun-1853	M	first child
Batten	Mrs. S.	2892	19-Apr-1857	M	third child
Batten	Mrs. S.	3318	08-Jan-1860	F	fourth child
Batter	Mrs. J. O.	3549	04-Aug-1861	F	fifth child
Batton	Mrs. S.	2519	30-Nov-1854	M	second child, attended by Dr Gibson
Baugher	Mrs. Constantine	2393	07-Feb-1854	M	first child
Baugher	Mrs. Constantine	2596	15-May-1855	F	second child
Baugher	Mrs. Constantine	2845	20-Dec-1856	F	third child
Baugher	Mrs. J. C.	3612	01-Feb-1862	F	fifth child
Baugher	Mrs. J. C.	4118	14-Jul-1866	F	fifth pregnancy
Baugher	Mrs. J.	3230	09-May-1859	M	fourth child
Bauskett	Mrs. J.	4265	21-Oct-1867	F	second pregnancy
Bauskett	Mrs. J.	4623	13-Dec-1870	M	fourth pregnancy

13

Obstetrical Casebooks of Dr. F. E. Chatard – an alternative genealogical resource 1829-1883

Bauskett	Mrs. John	4407	13-Jan-1869	F	third pregnancy
Bauskett	Mrs. John	4806	17-Dec-1872	M	fifth pregnancy, beginning ninth month, assisted "by my son." Child gave no signs of life
Bayless	Mrs. John	4370	06-Sep-1868	M	first pregnancy
Bazire	Mrs. A.	867	20-Jul-1843	M	second child
Beacham	Mrs.	1524	07-Jan-1848	F	born about 11:50 PM
Beatty	Mrs.	107	14-Jun-1834	M	third child
Beatty	Mrs.	466	29-Feb-1840	F	third child
Beatty	Mrs.	883	28-Aug-1843	F	fourth child
Beatty	Mrs. J.	426	27-Oct-1839	M	fourth child
Beatty	Mrs. James	2322	19-Aug-1853	F	first child
Beatty	Mrs. James	2673	26-Oct-1855	F	second child
Beatty	Mrs. James	2939	16-Jul-1857	F	third child
Beatty	Mrs. W.	3486	06-Feb-1861	F	fourth child
Beatty	Mrs. Wm.	3077	27-Apr-1858	M	third child
Beatty	Mrs. Wm.	3894	31-May-1864	M	fifth pregnancy
Beatty	Mrs. Wm.	3894	31-May-1864	M	fifth pregnancy
Beauchamp	Mrs.	1861	06-Jul-1850	F	fifth child
Bee	Mrs.	2788	01-Sep-1856	M	first child
Belknap	Mrs. Charles	4881	26-Jan-1874	M	first pregnancy, required morphine
Bell	Mrs.	368	02-Mar-1839	M	attended by Dr Perkins, still born
Bell	Mrs.	515	06-Aug-1840	F	(see #368), sixth child, still born
Bell	Mrs.	686	19-Feb-1842	M	seventh child, died during birth
Bell	Mrs.	2152	06-Jul-1852	F	second child
Bell	Mrs. J. S.	4810	13-Jan-1873	M	first pregnancy
Bell	Mrs. J. S.	5001	31-Aug-1875	F	third pregnancy

14

Obstetrical Casebooks of Dr. F. E. Chatard – an alternative genealogical resource 1829-1883

Bell	Mrs. Lizzie	4767	15-Jul-1872	F	first pregnancy
Bell	Mrs. Mary	2042	20-Oct-1851	F	second child
Bell	Mrs. Mary Ann	1501	25-Nov-1847	M	first child
Bell	Mrs. Sprigg	4216	02-May-1867	F	second pregnancy
Bell	Mrs. Wm.	674	18-Jan-1842	M	second child
Bell	Mrs. Wm.	2566	11-Mar-1855	F	first child
Belt	Mrs. Sprigg	3766	07-Apr-1863	M	first pregnancy
Bendann	Mrs. D.	4046	03-Nov-1865	F	first pregnancy
Bendann	Mrs. D.	4328	01-May-1868	F	third pregnancy
Bennett	Mrs. Adolphus	2667	06-Oct-1855	M	first child
Bennett	Mrs. Adolphus	3721	20-Dec-1862	M	second child
Bennett	Mrs. Adolphus	3976	21-Jan-1865	F	third pregnancy
Bennett	Mrs. Thomas S.	2931	06-Jul-1857	M	first child, attended by Dr. Yates, forceps
Berg	Mrs. A.	5121	09-May-1877	M	seventh pregnancy
Bernal	Mrs. Frdk	3533	14-Jun-1861	M	third child, lived but 36 hours
Berney	Mrs. James	2733	06-Apr-1855	M	ninth child
Berry	Mrs.	1573	05-May-1848	F	fourth child
Berry	Mrs.	1963	16-Mar-1851	F	fourth child
Berry	Mrs. J. T.	3546	21-Jul-1861	M	fourth child
Berry	Mrs. Jasper M.	2517	28-Nov-1854	M	first child
Berry	Mrs. Jasper M.	3215	20-Mar-1859	M	third child
Berry	Mrs. John	2929	03-Jul-1857	M	second child
Berry	Mrs. John	3168	01-Dec-1858	F	third child
Berry	Mrs. W. W.	2460	12-Aug-1854	F	fifth child
Berry	Mrs. Walter W.	2997	12-Nov-1857	M	seventh child
Betts	Mrs. E.	2787	31-Aug-1856	M	third child

15

Obstetrical Casebooks of Dr. F. E. Chatard – an alternative genealogical resource 1829-1883

Bettzhorn	Mrs. Elizabeth	2391	05-Feb-1854	F	fourth child
Bevan	Mrs.	33	07-Nov-1831		two months pregnant
Bevan	Mrs.	63	24-Jan-1833	M	see 7 Nov 1831 [#33]; sixth child, nine lbs.
Bevan	Mrs. J. S.	3774	26-Apr-1863	M	third pregnancy
Bevan	Mrs. John	3426	09-Oct-1860	M	second child
Bevan	Mrs. Joseph	534	16-Oct-1840	M	sixth child, stillborn
Bevan	Mrs. William	2145	06-Jun-1852	F	first child
Bevan	Mrs. Wm. J.	2324	23-Aug-1853	M	second child
Birch	Mrs. C.	4855	18-Sep-1873	F	first pregnancy
Bird	Mrs. Edward	1522	02-Jan-1848	M	first child
Bird	Mrs. Edward	2071	13-Dec-1851	F	third child
Bird	Mrs. J. Conrad	3838	13-Jan-1864	M	sixth pregnancy
Bird	Mrs. J. Edward	1722	09-Jul-1849	F	second child
Bird	Mrs. J. Edward	2490	30-Sep-1854	F	fourth child
Bird	Mrs. J. Edward	2942	27-Jul-1857	M	fifth child
Bird	Mrs. J. Edward	3362	03-May-1860	M	sixth child
Bird	Mrs. Joseph A.	3271	12-Sep-1859	M	first child
Biscoe	Mrs.	911	28-Oct-1843	F	born 6:15 PM
Bitterbaugh	Mrs. George	117	09-Sep-1834	M	second child, violent convulsions
Bizonard	Madame	9	M		third child, "Expected to be delivered by my father, was so startled by seeing me that pains left her."
Blacklick	Mrs. F.	759	11-Sep-1842		second child
Blacklick	Mrs. N. F.	1133	28-Feb-1845	M	third child
Blacklick	Mrs. N. F.	2349	07-Nov-1853	M	first child
Blacklock	Mrs.	570	26-Jan-1841	F	first child

16

Obstetrical Casebooks of Dr. F. E. Chatard – an alternative genealogical resource 1829-1883

Blair	Mrs.	849	16-May-1845	M	sixth child
Blair	Mrs.	1044	24-Sep-1844	M	seventh child
Blinsinger	Mrs. George	2424	17-May-1854	M	second child
Blinsinger	Mrs. George	3305	13-Dec-1859	M	third child
Blinsinger	Mrs. Mary	2148	17-Jun-1852	F	born 4 PM
Blum	Mrs. S.	4577	27-Jul-1870	F	eighth pregnancy
Blundell	Mrs. Anthony	2174	07-Sep-1852	M	third child
Bodewin	Mrs. Charles	5076	14-Aug-1876	F	first pregnancy
Bogue	Mrs.	432	07-Nov-1839	F	second child
Bogue	Mrs. H.	276	02-Jan-1837	F	first child
Bogue	Mrs. Henry	1656	27-Dec-1848	M	seventh child
Bogue	Mrs. Henry	1766	21-Oct-1849	F	eighth child
Bogue	Mrs. John	1285	27-May-1846	M	second child
Bogue	Mrs. Robert	5050	15-Apr-1876	F	first pregnancy
Bogue	Mrs. Robert	5144	22-Aug-1877	M	second pregnancy
Bogue	Mrs. Robert	5175	07-Dec-1873	M	third pregnancy
Bogue	Mrs. Robert	5239	20-Jul-1881	F/F	fourth pregnancy
Boice	Mrs. G.	1298	26-Jun-1846	F	second child
Boker	Mrs. B. H.	4467	20-Jul-1869	M	first pregnancy
Böker	Mrs. B. H.	4667	28-May-1871	F	second pregnancy
Böker	Mrs. B. H.	4813	29-Jan-1873	M	third pregnancy
Bolling	Mrs. W.	4650	13-Apr-1871	M	first pregnancy
Bolling	Mrs. W. N.	5009	07-Oct-1875	F	third pregnancy
Bolling	Mrs. W.N.	5211	17-Dec-1879	F	fifth pregnancy, patient attended by Dr. Bowie
Bonaparte	Mrs. Jerome N.	1983	09-Jun-1851	M	second child. Her first child was born in 1830 about one year after her marriage consequently nearly 21 years have elapsed between the two

17

Obstetrical Casebooks of Dr. F. E. Chatard – an alternative genealogical resource 1829-1883

					births.
Bond	Mrs. H. L.	2660	27-Sep-1855	M	first child
Bond	Mrs. Hugh L.	3177	23-Dec-1858	M	second child
Bondon	Mrs.	739	28-Jul-1842	M	first child
Bonie	Mrs. H. Ray	1144	30-Apr-1845	F	second child
Bonninger	Mrs.	1130	19-Feb-1845	F	second child
Bonninger	Mrs. G.	863	05-Jul-1843	M	born 2:45 PM
Bonninger	Mrs. G.	1357	26-Nov-1846	M	third child
Boone	Mrs. W.	4548	13-May-1870	M	third pregnancy
Boone	Mrs. W.	4776	29-Aug-1872	F	fifth pregnancy
Boone	Mrs. W.	4948	02-Nov-1874	F	seventh pregnancy, eight months, "… had a severe fright two days previous and was seen & prescribed for by Dr J. Jenkins. Taken with severe convulsions …" stillborn
Boone	Mrs. Wm.	4366	25-Aug-1868	M	second pregnancy
Boone	Mrs. Wm.	4869	21-Dec-1873	F	sixth pregnancy
Boone	Mrs. Wm. M.	4171	28-Dec-1866	F	first pregnancy
Bordley	Mrs. J.	4962	11-Dec-1874	F	fourth pregnancy
Boreland	Mrs.	1526	13-Jan-1848	M	assisted by Dr Hintze
Bostick	Mrs. Maria	2050	06-Nov-1851	F	first child, difficult birth, child died
Boston	Mrs.	390	09-Jun-1839	F	second child
Boston	Mrs.	623	12-Aug-1841	M	third child
Boston	Mrs.	1489	11-Oct-1847	M	sixth child
Boston	Mrs. J. B.	1234	04-Dec-1845	M	fifth child
Botoce [?]	Mrs. Helen	1078	24-Nov-1844	M	first child
Bottimore	Mrs. F.	1196	24-Aug-1845	M	third child
Bottimore	Mrs. F.	1447	21-Jun-1847	F	fourth child

Obstetrical Casebooks of Dr. F. E. Chatard – an alternative genealogical resource 1829-1883

Bottimore	Mrs. Frederick	2133	16-May-1852	M	fifth child
Bottimore	Mrs. Frederick	2423	14-May-1854	F	born 4:45 AM
Bottimore	Mrs. Fredk.	788	05-Dec-1842	M	second child
Bottimore	Mrs. Thomas	2035	10-Oct-1851	F	first child
Bottomer	Mrs. Harry H.	5020	30-Nov-1875	M	second pregnancy
Bottonere [?]	Mrs. Henry	4942	05-Oct-1874	F	first pregnancy
Boucher	Mrs. W.	4775	28-Aug-1872	F	fifth pregnancy
Boucher	Mrs. William	5198	08-Aug-1879	F	tenth pregnancy
Boucher	Mrs. William	5229	05-Dec-1880	M	11th pregnancy
Boucher	Mrs. Wm.	4863	23-Oct-1873	F	sixth pregnancy
Boucher, Jr.	Mrs. W.	5051	19-Apr-1876	M	eighth pregnancy, "The child was nearly asphyxiated & was brought to after considerable manipulation."
Boucher, Jr.	Mrs. William	5132	23-Jun-1877	M	ninth pregnancy
Boucher, Jr.	Mrs. Wm.	4968	07-Jan-1875	F	seventh pregnancy
Boucher, Jr.	Mrs. Wm.	5248	03-Mar-1882	F	12th pregnancy
Boudoin	Mrs. S. L.	781	24-Nov-1842	F	fifth child
Bourand	Mrs.	667	02-Jan-1842	F	second child
Bourbeau	Mrs. August	4187	06-Feb-1867	F	fourth pregnancy
Bourne	Mrs. George	3605	12-Jan-1862	M	fifth child
Bourne	Mrs. P. Arell	3852	04-Feb-1864	M	second pregnancy
Boursand	Madame	904	15-Oct-1843	F	third child
Boursand	Mrs.	1230	19-Nov-1845	F	fourth child. This lady on the 22d October fell while standing on a small ladder which shifted from under her. The knee was cut severely … and was still suppurating freely
Boursand	Mrs.	1424	20-Apr-1847	F	fifth child
Boursand	Mrs.	1789	19-Dec-1849	M	sixth child, died on 20th

Obstetrical Casebooks of Dr. F. E. Chatard – an alternative genealogical resource 1829-1883

Bowdoin	Mrs.	966	11-Mar-1844	F	second child
Bowdoin	Mrs. Severn	1107	24-Jan-1845	F	born 10 AM
Bowdoin	Mrs. Severn	1305	12-Jul-1846	M	born 7 AM
Bowdoin	Mrs. Severn	1665	25-Jan-1849	F	ninth child
Bowdoin	Mrs. Severn	2564	04-Mar-1855	F	11th child
Bowdoin	Mrs. Severn E.	1503	28-Nov-1847	M	eighth child
Bowdoin	Mrs. W. G.	5262	14-Jan-1883	F	third pregnancy, post partum complications.
Bowdoin	Mrs. William G.	5225	04-Oct-1880	M	second pregnancy
Bowerman	Mrs. R. N.	4037	05-Oct-1865	F	fifth pregnancy
Bowerman	Mrs. Richard	4279	14-Nov-1867	F	seventh pregnancy
Bowie	Mrs. Dr.	1244	31-Dec-1845	M	second child
Bowie	Mrs. Dr. A.	1549	05-Mar-1848	M	third child
Bowie	Mrs. H. R.	1277	02-May-1846	F	third child
Bowie	Mrs. Hyde R.	910	27-Oct-1843	M	first child
Bowley	Mrs. Daniel	970	19-Mar-1844	M	second child
Boyce	Mrs.	793	16-Dec-1842	M	first child, mother had virulent headache
Boyce	Mrs. James	1955	02-Mar-1851	M	first child
Boyce	Mrs. James	2290	07-Jun-1853	F	second child
Boyce	Mrs. James	2884	27-Mar-1857	F	third child
Boyce	Mrs. James	3478	19-Jan-1861	M	fifth child
Boyce	Mrs. James	3817	28-Oct-1863	M	seventh pregnancy
Boyd	Mrs.	31	22-Oct-1831	F	aged 20, first child, seven pounds
Boyd	Mrs.	187	08-May-1836	F	third child
Boyd	Mrs. Wm.	296	05-Apr-1838	M	fourth child weighed 9 pounds
Boyd	Mrs. Wm.	401	03-Aug-1839	M	fifth child
Boyd	Mrs. Wm.	545	23-Nov-1840	F	sixth child

Obstetrical Casebooks of Dr. F. E. Chatard – an alternative genealogical resource 1829-1883

Boyd	Mrs. Wm. A.	3385	22-Jun-1860	F	second child
Boyer	Caroline	487	08-May-1840	F	apparently twins, male died, female survived
Boyle	Mrs. James	4919	05-Aug-1874	F	seventh pregnancy
Bra....	Madame	882	26-Aug-183	F	fourth child
Bracher	Mrs. W.	4644	13-Feb-1871	M	fourth pregnancy, attended by Dr. McSherry. "The child was nearly lifeless & was recovered with great difficulty."
Brademyer	Mrs. Charles	3965	30-Dec-1864	M	second pregnancy, acephalic
Bradford	Mrs. J. Stricker	1118	07-Feb-1845		first child, stillborn
Bradford	Mrs. J. Stricker	1258	02-Feb-1846	M	second child
Brady	Mrs.	14	01-Jun-1830		first child
Brady	Mrs.	60	11-Dec-1832	M	see June 1830 [#14], second child
Brady	Mrs. Hugh	334	13-Sep-1838	M	first child
Brady	Mrs. Hugh	457	12-Jan-1840	M	second child
Brady	Mrs. Hugh	645	22-Oct-1841	F	fifth child
Brady	Mrs. Hugh	846	11-May-1843	M	fourth child
Brady	Mrs. Hugh	1071	06-Nov-1844	M	born 10:20 AM
Brady	Mrs. Hugh	1289	06-Jun-1846	F	Child being born when I arrived.
Brady	Mrs. Hugh	1472	28-Aug-1847	M	seventh child
Brady	Mrs. Hugh	1675	16-Feb-1849	M	eighth child
Brady	Mrs. Hugh	1842	17-May-1850	F	ninth child
Brady	Mrs. Hugh	2014	15-Aug-1851	F	born 4 PM
Brady	Mrs. Hugh	3017	12-Dec-1857	M	11th child
Brady	Mrs. James	765	01-Oct-1842	M	first child
Brady	Mrs. James	1062	23-Oct-1844	M	second child
Brady	Mrs. James	2913	11-Jun-1857	M	first child

Obstetrical Casebooks of Dr. F. E. Chatard – an alternative genealogical resource 1829-1883

Brady	Mrs. James	3260	06-Aug-1859	F	second child
Brady	Mrs. Philip	154	28-Jul-1835	M	see 11 Dec 1832 [#60], third child
Bragasse	Mrs. F.	3782	13-Jun-1863	M	first pregnancy
Brand	Mrs. A. J.	871	26-Jul-1843	M	first child
Brand	Mrs. A. J.	1124	14-Feb-1845	F	second child
Brandt	Mrs. Jacob	2414	26-Apr-1854	F	second child
Brandt	Mrs. Jacob	2619	15-Jul-1855	F	third child
Brandt	Mrs. Jacob	2781	13-Aug-1856	F	fourth child
Brandt	Mrs. Jacob	3029	03-Jan-1858	F	fifth child
Brandt	Mrs. Jacob	3237	21-May-1859	M	sixth child
Brandt	Mrs. Jacob	3420	25-Sep-1860	M	seventh child
Brandt	Mrs. Jacob	3834	01-Jan-1864	M	ninth pregnancy
Brandt	Mrs. Jacob	4066	28-Dec-1865	M	tenth pregnancy
Brandt	Mrs. Jacob	4348	08-Jul-1868	F	11th pregnancy
Brandt	Mrs. Jacob	4903	19-May-1874	F	12th pregnancy
Brannan	Mrs. Peter	3252	04-Jul-1859	M	tenth child
Brannan	Mrs. Peter	3848	25-Jan-1864	M	11th pregnancy
Brehm	Mrs. O.	4731	08-Jan-1872	F	eighth pregnancy
Brehme	Mrs. O.	3711	01-Dec-1862	M	second child, attended by Dr. Chew
Brehme	Mrs. O.	3925	20-Sep-1864	M	third pregnancy
Brehme	Mrs. O.	4232	05-Jul-1867	F	fifth pregnancy
Brehme	Mrs. O.	4474	06-Aug-1869	M	sixth pregnancy
Brehme	Mrs. O.	4607	05-Nov-1870	F/M	seventh pregnancy, twins 8.5 and 9.5 pounds
Brehme	Mrs. O.	5047	03-Apr-1876	M	ninth pregnancy. "She was much exhausted by the labours … the head was large & the child of considerable size."
Brehme	Mrs. O.	5193	06-Jun-1879	F/F	tenth pregnancy, eight months, twins

Obstetrical Casebooks of Dr. F. E. Chatard – an alternative genealogical resource 1829-1883

Breline [Brehine]	Mrs. O.	4041	12-Oct-1865	M	fourth pregnancy
Brenan	Mrs. F. H.	3468	21-Dec-1860	F	fourth child
Brenan	Mrs. F. X.	3995	22-Apr-1865	M	fifth pregnancy
Brenan	Mrs. Francis	2280	12-May-1853	F	first child
Brenan	Mrs. Francis	2559	19-Feb-1855	M	second held
Brenan	Mrs. O.	2661	29-Sep-1855	M	first child
Brenan	Mrs. Oliver	2956	03-Sep-1857		second child
Brenan	Mrs. Oliver	3276	26-Sep-1859	M	third child
Brenan	Mrs. Oliver	3696	30-Oct-1862	M	fourth child
Brevar [?]	Mrs. Francis X.	3809	30-Aug-1863	F	fifth pregnancy
Brickhead	Mrs. John	4277	08-Nov-1867	F	first pregnancy, attended by Drs. Henry & Hopkins. "She died a few days after."
Bridener	Mrs. George M.	5183	13-Mar-1879	M	third pregnancy
Bridge	Mrs. Margaret	2201	07-Nov-1852	F	first child
Brien	Mrs. John	663	08-Dec-1841	F	sixth child
Bright	Mrs.	1924	06-Dec-1850	M	first child
Bright	Mrs. Henry	2180	14-Sep-1852	F	second child
Bright	Mrs. Henry	2498	13-Oct-1854	M	third child, premature, stillborn
Briscoe	Mrs.	531	14-Oct-1840	F	third child
Briscoe	Mrs.	1387	29-Jan-1847		fifth child
Briscoe	Mrs. S. W.	3954	07-Dec-1864	F	first pregnancy
Broadbent	Mrs. Stephen	662	04-Dec-1841	F	fifth child
Brodherton	Mrs. David H.	5200	10-Sep-1879	M	first pregnancy, forceps delivery. "The child became asphyxiated could not be made to breath."
Brodmeyer	Mrs.	220	14-Jan-1837	F	second child

Obstetrical Casebooks of Dr. F. E. Chatard – an alternative genealogical resource 1829-1883

Brooks	Mrs. John	684	01-Feb-1842	M	fifth child
Broughton	Mrs. J.	2444	07-Jul-1854	M	first child. "Attended by a midwife during my absence."
Brove	Mrs. J. I.	4315	16-Mar-1868	M	fifth pregnancy
Brown	Mrs. T. M.	4416	07-Feb-1869	M	first pregnancy
Brown	Mrs.	510	19-Jul-1840		first child
Brown	Mrs.	1363	05-Dec-1846	F	fifth child
Brown	Mrs. Albert M.	3175	19-Dec-1858	F	third child
Brown	Mrs. C. H. H.	311	10-Jul-1838	M	second child
Brown	Mrs. C. H. H.	656	15-Nov-1841	M	fourth child
Brown	Mrs. Dr. G.	3828	06-Dec-1863	F	second child
Brown	Mrs. Dr. T. R.	4541	07-May-1870	F	first pregnancy
Brown	Mrs. George	2494	08-Oct-1854	M	first child
Brown	Mrs. George	2694	23-Dec-1855	F	second child
Brown	Mrs. George	4306	13-Feb-1868	F	(of Alex.), first pregnancy
Brown	Mrs. George	4463	07-Jul-1869	F	second pregnancy
Brown	Mrs. George	4597	17-Oct-1870	M	third pregnancy
Brown	Mrs. George	4629	04-Jan-1871	F	fourth pregnancy
Brown	Mrs. George	4757	01-Jun-1872	F	fourth pregnancy
Brown	Mrs. George W.	1053	15-Oct-1844		third child
Brown	Mrs. J. S.	123	07-Nov-1834		abortion of about six weeks
Brown	Mrs. J. W.	3610	29-Jan-1862	M	first child
Brown	Mrs. J. Wilson	4839	17-Jun-1873	F	sixth pregnancy
Brown	Mrs. J. Wilson	5006	28-Sep-1875	F	seventh pregnancy
Brown	Mrs. Robert	4222	29-May-1867	F	third pregnancy
Brown	Mrs. T. J.	2023	02-Sep-1851	M	third child

Obstetrical Casebooks of Dr. F. E. Chatard – an alternative genealogical resource 1829-1883

Browne	Mrs. A. P.	4471	31-Jul-1869	F	sixth pregnancy
Browne	Mrs. Arrell P.	4176	19-Jan-1867	F	fourth pregnancy
Browne	Mrs. P. A.	4323	11-Apr-1868	M	fifth pregnancy
Browne	Mrs. P. Arroll	5127	14-Jun-1877	F	tenth pregnancy
Browne	Mrs. P. Asnell	4888	03-Mar-1874	F	eighth pregnancy
Browne	Mrs. Peter Arnold	5045	19-Mar-1876	F	ninth pregnancy
Bruce	Mrs.	4109	22-Jun-1866	F	fourth pregnancy, "was attacked with convulsions about six weeks before…" Child stillborn
Brun	Mad. F.	1975	11-May-1851	M	seventh child
Brun	Madame	1634	18-Oct-1848	M/	born 10 PM, twins
Brun	Mrs. E.	4689	10-Aug-1871	F	first pregnancy, "natural but tedious, the case in charge of my son."
Brun	Mrs. Edward	4938	26-Sep-1874	M	second pregnancy, forceps delivery
Brun	Mrs. F.	633	19-Sep-1841	M	third child
Brun	Mrs. Francis	394	08-Jul-1839	F	second child
Brundige	Mrs. W.	514	04-Aug-1840	M	stillborn
Brundt	Mrs. Carlos	2570	20-Mar-1855	F	second child
Brune	Mrs. P. Arrell	4014	18-Jun-1865	F	third pregnancy
Brunet	Mrs. Carlos	2285	26-May-1853	M	second child
Bruns [?]	Mrs. Arrell	3645	04-Jun-1862	M	first child
Brunst	Mrs. Carlos	2920	18-Jun-1857	M	fourth child
Buchanan	Mrs. James M.	135	01-Feb-1835	M	second child
Buchannan	Mrs. J.	241	02-Jul-1837	M	third child
Buchannan	Mrs. James M.	2370	25-Dec-1853	F	ninth child
Buchannan	Mrs. V. H.	3963	29-Dec-1864	F	first pregnancy
Buchannon	Mrs. J. M.	351	24-Nov-1838	F	fourth child

Obstetrical Casebooks of Dr. F. E. Chatard – an alternative genealogical resource 1829-1883

Buchannon	Mrs. James	1405	17-Mar-1847	F	seventh child
Buchannon	Mrs. James M.	589	24-Apr-1841	M	fifth child
Buchannon	Mrs. James M.	929	09-Dec-1843	M	sixth child
Buchannon	Mrs. James M.	1802	26-Jan-1850	M	born 8:20 AM
Buck	Mrs. John M.	1031	30-Aug-1844	F	fourth child
Buckler	Mrs. Dr. Riggin	4310	01-Mar-1868	F	sixth pregnancy
Buffington	Mrs. Levi	3550	06-Aug-1861	F	11th child
Bulkely	Mrs.	162	27-Oct-1835	F	first child
Bumap	Mrs. G. W.	698	28-Mar-1842	F	third child
Burke	Mrs. J. M.	4529	27-Feb-1870	M	first pregnancy
Burke	Mrs. J. M.	4690	16-Aug-1871	M	second pregnancy
Burke	Mrs. John	3541	09-Jul-1861	F	first child, forceps delivery
Burnes	Mrs. Dr. Arthur	3649	14-Jun-1862	F	eight months
Burns	Mrs.	2101	17-Feb-1852	F	ninth child
Burns	Mrs. A. P.	2967	21-Sep-1857	F	fifth child
Burns	Mrs. Andrew	1153	17-May-1845	M	first child
Burns	Mrs. Dr. Arthur P.	1871	05-Aug-1850	M	first child
Burns	Mrs. J.	4468	20-Jul-1869		first pregnancy, stillborn
Burns	Mrs. J.	4736	28-Feb-1872	F	fourth pregnancy, eight months, "All the patient's children have been premature."
Burns	Mrs. John	4552	25-May-1870	M/F	second pregnancy, attended by Dr. Stevenson, twins, both died
Burns	Mrs. Pierce	3589	14-Nov-1861	F	assisted by Dr. VanBibber
Burns	Mrs. R. D.	370	09-Mar-1839	F	fifth child
Burns	Mrs. R. D.	744	07-Aug-1842	F	six months, born dead

26

Obstetrical Casebooks of Dr. F. E. Chatard – an alternative genealogical resource 1829-1883

Burns	Mrs. R. D.	889	10-Sep-1843	F	six months
Burns	Mrs. Robert	4121	25-Jul-1866	F	first pregnancy
Burns	Mrs. Robert	4349	08-Jul-1868	F	second pregnancy
Burrow	Mrs. F. M.	4336	22-May-1858	M	third pregnancy
Burrow	Mrs. F. N.	4127	30-Jul-1866	M	second pregnancy
Buschman	Mrs. V. H.	4140	29-Aug-1866	F	second pregnancy
Byrne	Mrs. E.	1268	28-Mar-1846	F	third child
Byrne	Mrs. E. H.	1551	11-Mar-1848	M	fourth child
Byrne	Mrs. Edward	1151	16-May-1845	M	second child
Byrne	Mrs. Edward H.	1853	23-Jun-1850	F	fifth child
Byrne	Mrs. Edward H.	2278	11-May-1853	F	sixth child
Byrne	Mrs. H.	4617	05-Dec-1870	F	third pregnancy
C.[hatard]	Mrs.	128	13-Dec-1834	M	see 27 Jan 1833 [#65], second child, eight lbs.
C.[hatard]	Mrs.	213	29-Oct-1836	M	third child
C[hatard]	Mrs.	65	27-Jan-1833	F	first child, 8.25 pounds
C[hatard]	Mrs.	616	31-Jul-1841	F	fifth child
C[hatard]	Mrs. F.	1157	22-May-1845	M	seventh child
Caffray	Mrs.	48	18-Jul-1832	M	third child
Caldwell	Mrs. James	1092	27-Dec-1844	F	first child
Callum	Mrs. Nelson	1484	29-Sep-1847	M	second child
Calvert	Mrs. Susan	2656	19-Sep-1855	M	colored, third child
Calvert	Mrs. Susan	3324	13-Jan-1860	M	colored, fifth child
Calvert	Susan	2003	17-Jul-1851	M	colored. First child
Calvert	Susan	2325	23-Aug-1853	F	colored, second child
Calvert	Susan	2952	23-Aug-1857	F	colored, fourth child
Calvert	Susan	3904	13-Jul-1864	F	colored, sixth pregnancy

Obstetrical Casebooks of Dr. F. E. Chatard – an alternative genealogical resource 1829-1883

Campbell	Mrs. B. J.	4498	29-Oct-1869	M	second pregnancy
Campbell	Mrs. J.	721	26-May-1842	M	second child
Campbell	Mrs. Peter	4497	27-Oct-1869	F	seventh pregnancy
Cansell	Mrs. J. F.	2415	27-Apr-1854	F	first child
Carey	Mrs.	1971	30-Apr-1851	M	third child
Carey	Mrs. Henry G.	4130	09-Aug-1866	M	first pregnancy
Carey	Mrs. John	3174	16-Dec-1858	M	second child
Carey	Mrs. Thomas	5015	01-Nov-1875	M	fourth pregnancy, "labour slow & difficult. All her labours were of the same character she told me & all were terminated with forceps."
Carland	Mrs.	19	11-Nov-1830		fourth child
Carland	Mrs.	55	02-Oct-1832	F	see 15 Nov 1830 [#19]; fifth child
Carland	Mrs.	115	04-Sep-1834	M	see 2 Oct 1832 [#55], sixth child, 10.5 lbs.
Carlett	Mrs. William	3075	21-Apr-1858	M	first child
Carman	Mrs.	3929	26-Sep-1864	F	first pregnancy
Carman	Mrs. J. D.	4961	07-Dec-1874	M	fourth pregnancy
Carman	Mrs. Joseph D.	4180	25-Jan-1867	M	second pregnancy
Carman	Mrs. Joseph D.	4637	20-Jan-1871	M	third pregnancy
Carpanteur	Mrs. Rosa	1494	20-Oct-1847	M	sixth child
Carpenter	Mrs. W. C.	1819	19-Feb-1850	M	first child
Carpenter	Mrs. W. C.	2011	10-Aug-1851	M	second child
Carr	Mrs. H. K.	2875	07-Mar-1857	M	attended by Dr. Ed. Baker, child died next day
Carr	Mrs. J.	4879	18-Jan-1874	F	third pregnancy
Carr	Mrs. James	1827	13-Mar-1850	M	first child, The child though apparently healthy died within the course of the day.
Carr	Mrs. James	3840	13-Jan-1864	F	sixth pregnancy

28

Carr	Mrs. James	4734	27-Jan-1872	M	eighth pregnancy, attended by a midwife, child was dead
Carr	Mrs. John	2936	13-Jul-1857	F	first child
Carr	Mrs. John	3156	03-Nov-1858	F	second child
Carr	Mrs. Nicholas	2160	27-Jul-1852	F	second child
Carr	Mrs. Nicholas	2630	10-Aug-1855	F	third child
Carr	Mrs. Nicholas	3042	08-Feb-1858	M	fifth child
Carr	Mrs. Nicholas	3462	12-Dec-1860	M	sixth child
Carr	Mrs. R. Wilson	2318	08-Aug-1853	M	born 8:15 AM. "Per her request, I gave her chloroform with … She was not conscious of the birth of the child."
Carrington	Mrs. J. K.	751	25-Aug-1842	F	first child
Carrington	Mrs. J. K.	1066	27-Oct-1844	F	second child
Carrington	Mrs. J. K.	1366	15-Dec-1846	M	third child
Carroll	Mrs. John	3684	23-Sep-1862	M	third child
Carroll	Mrs. John	4084	19-Feb-1866	F	first pregnancy
Carroll	Mrs. Albert	3195	06-Feb-1859	F	first child
Carroll	Mrs. Albert	3457	07-Dec-1860	F	second child
Carroll	Mrs. Albert	3735	15-Jan-1863	F	third child
Carroll	Mrs. C. Tucker	3927	21-Sep-1864	M	second pregnancy
Carroll	Mrs. C. Tucker	4345	24-Jun-1868	M	third pregnancy
Carroll	Mrs. Charles R.	477	04-Apr-1840	F	10th child
Carroll	Mrs. Charles R.	664	10-Dec-1841	M	born 1:20 AM
Carroll	Mrs. Charles R.	868	21-Jul-1843	F	tenth child
Carroll	Mrs. Charles R.	1047	08-Oct-1844	F	13th child
Carroll	Mrs. Henry P.	3638	19-May-1862	F	sixth child
Carroll	Mrs. J. N.	4769	17-Jul-1872	M	second pregnancy
Carroll	Mrs. James	1576	13-May-1848	F	sixth child

Obstetrical Casebooks of Dr. F. E. Chatard – an alternative genealogical resource 1829-1883

Carroll	Mrs. John	3435	28-Oct-1860	M	second child
Carroll	Mrs. John	5022	08-Dec-1875	F	second pregnancy, consultation with Dr Janney, child dead
Carroll	Mrs. John Lee	3971	12-Jan-1865	M	fifth pregnancy
Carroll	Mrs. John N.	4646	04-Mar-1871	M	first pregnancy
Carroll	Mrs. Mary Ann	3228	06-May-1859	F	first child
Carroll	Mrs. Mortimer	3814	04-Oct-1863	M	first pregnancy
Carroll	Mrs. Mortimer	4152	13-Oct-1866	F	third pregnancy
Carroll	Mrs. Mortimore	3988	05-Apr-1865	M	second pregnancy
Carroll	Mrs. S. J.	2136	25-May-1852	F	second child
Carroll	Mrs. Wm.	953	24-Jan-1844	M	fourth child
Carroll	Mrs. Wm. P.	3765	06-Apr-1863	M	first pregnancy. "…had been & was still suffering under a severe attack of Rheumatism."
Carroll, Jr.	Mrs. James	316	22-Jul-1838	M	first child
Carroll, Jr.	Mrs. James	523	19-Sep-1840	F	second child
Carroll, Jr.	Mrs. James	659	27-Nov-1841	M	third child
Carroll, Jr.	Mrs. James	840	20-Apr-1843	M	fourth child
Carroll, Jr.	Mrs. James	1237	07-Dec-1845	M	fifth child
Carroll, Jr.	Mrs. James	1900	15-Oct-1850	M	seventh child
Carson	Mrs. John	727	26-Jun-1842	F	second child
Carson	Mrs. John	891	18-Sep-1843	F	third child
Carson	Mrs. T. J.	1442	06-Jun-1847	F	second child
Carson	Mrs. Thomas J.	1867	31-Jul-1850	M	third child
Carter	Mrs. Bernard	4641	03-Feb-1871	M	tenth pregnancy
Carter	Mrs. C.	4530	07-Mar-1870	F	third pregnancy
Carter	Mrs. Charles	3843	15-Jan-1864	M	first pregnancy
Carter	Mrs. Charles	4067	28-Dec-1865	M	second pregnancy

Obstetrical Casebooks of Dr. F. E. Chatard – an alternative genealogical resource 1829-1883

Carter	Mrs. Charles	4815	18-Feb-1873	M	fourth pregnancy
Carver	Mrs.	1779	28-Nov-1849	M	second child
Carver	Mrs. W. V.	3942	06-Nov-1864	F	eight pregnancy
Carver	Mrs. W. V.	4274	31-Oct-1867	M	ninth pregnancy, child dead
Carver	Mrs. W. V.	4958	01-Dec-1874	F	12th pregnancy
Carver	Mrs. William	2860	09-Feb-1857	M	fifth child
Carver	Mrs. William	3234	14-May-1859	M	sixth child
Carver	Mrs. Wm	2147	13-Jun-1852	F	third child
Carver	Mrs. Wm.	2480	18-Sep-1854	F	fourth child
Carver	Mrs. Wm. V.	3603	05-Jan-1862	M	seventh child
Carver	Mrs. Wm. V.	4570	10-Jul-1870	M	tenth pregnancy
Carvill	Mrs. Wm.	1500	23-Nov-1847	F	first child
Carville	Mrs. Henry	1263	25-Feb-1846	F	second child
Carville	Mrs. Henry	1462	10-Aug-47	M	third child
Cary	Mrs. Wm.	2558	17-Feb-1855	M	fifth child
Casey	Mrs.	1514	18-Dec-1847	M	first child
Casey	Mrs.	1723	12-Jul-1849	M	second child
Casey	Mrs. Thomas	3701	06-Nov-1862	M	first child
Casey	Mrs. W.	1259	05-Feb-1846	F	first child
Casey	Mrs. Wm.	2237	02-Feb-1853	M	fourth child
Casey	Mrs. Wm.	2868	28-Feb-1857	F	sixth child
Cassard	Mrs. John	2886	02-Apr-1857	F	first child, breech, child died, mother died at 7:30PM
Cassell	Mrs. C.	4771	22-Jul-1872	M	second pregnancy
Cassell	Mrs. C. C.	5098	19-Jan-1877	F	fifth pregnancy
Cassell	Mrs. Charles	4614	03-Dec-1870	F	first pregnancy
Cassell	Mrs. Charles	4894	30-Mar-1874	F	third pregnancy

Obstetrical Casebooks of Dr. F. E. Chatard – an alternative genealogical resource 1829-1883

Cassell	Mrs. Charles E.	5002	02-Sep-1875	M	fourth pregnancy
Cassidy	Mrs. Francis	3241	25-May-1859	M	first child
Cassidy	Mrs. Francis	3471	27-Dec-1860	M	second child
Cassidy	Mrs. Francis	4898	19-Apr-1874	M	eighth pregnancy
Cassidy	Mrs. Francis	5068	19-Jul-1876	F	ninth pregnancy
Cassidy	Mrs. J.	1245	02-Jan-1846	F	second child
Cassidy	Mrs. J.	1987	14-Jun-1851	F	fourth child
Cassidy	Mrs. James	1012	10-Jul-1844	F	first child
Cassidy	Mrs. James	1639	02-Nov-1848	F	third child
Cassidy	Mrs. M.	2891	18-Apr-1857	M	fifth child
Cassidy	Mrs. Patrick	1713	03-Jun-1849	M	first child, died after first breath
Caughy	Mrs. Charles M.	5230	10-Jan-1881	M	first pregnancy
Cavalier	Mrs. G. P. M.	4313	11-Mar-1868	M	first pregnancy
Cavanagh	Mrs. Peter	3034	12-Jan-1858	M	second child
Cellans	Mrs. John	1970	23-Apr-1851	M	second child
Cercille	Josephine	35	26-Nov-1831	F	16 years old, colored, first child; five pounds. "She walked about a half a mile twenty four hours after delivery."
Chalk	Mrs. James	3706	16-Nov-1862	M	fourth child
Chalmers	Mrs.	212	29-Oct-1836		attended by two other physicians, "I found her exceedingly debilitated & prostate." Child dead. "The mother sunk rapidly & died about one hour after being delivered."
Chamberlain	Mrs.	741	01-Aug-1842	F	first child
Chamberlain	Mrs.	1699	06-Apr-1849		fourth child, stillborn
Chamberlin	Mrs.	1400	06-Mar-1847	F	third child
Chandler	Mrs. G. H.	4700	21-Oct-1871	F	first pregnancy

Obstetrical Casebooks of Dr. F. E. Chatard – an alternative genealogical resource 1829-1883

Chandler	Mrs. G. H.	4875	01-Jan-1874	F	second pregnancy
Chandler	Mrs. George	5016	13-Nov-75	M/	third pregnancy, twins, second child dead. Mother died on 8th day
Chandonet	Mrs. Antony	4933	14-Sep-1874	F	seventh pregnancy, "… the pains were very violent."
Chaney	Mrs. Floyd	2081	07-Jan-1852	F	second child
Chanson	Mrs. F.	1111	27-Jan-1845	M	second child
Chanson	Mrs. Francis	923	25-Nov-1843	F	first child
Chapell	Mrs. S. M.	2921	18-Jun-1857	M	second child
Chapin	Mrs. Philip	360	28-Jan-1839	M	first child
Chapin	Mrs. Philip	755	31-Aug-1842	M	second child
Chapin	Mrs. Philip	1113	30-Jan-1845	F	third child
Chapin	Mrs. Philip	1486	30-Sep-1847	F	fourth child
Chapin	Mrs. Philip	1839	07-May-1850	M	fifth child
Chapin	Mrs. Philip	2255	15-Mar-1853	M	sixth child
Chapin	Mrs. Philip	2670	15-Oct-1855	M	seventh child
Chapman	Mrs. Jonathan	3323	11-Jan-1860	M	sixth child
Chapman	Mrs. Jonathan	3844	15-Jan-1864	M	eighth pregnancy
Chapman	Mrs. Jonathan J.	3622	17-Mar-1862	M	seventh child
Chapman	Mrs. N. P.	3284	20-Oct-1859	F	third child
Chappell	Mrs. S. M.	3361	22-Apr-1860	M	fourth child
Chappell	Mrs. Samuel M.	3102	26-Jul-1858	F	third child
Charron	Mrs. J. B.	697	26-Mar-1842	F	first child
Charron	Mrs. J. B.	957	07-Feb-1844	M	born 4 AM
Charron	Mrs. J. B.	1256	02-Feb-1846	M	third child
Charron	Mrs. J. B.	1532	01-Jan-1848	M	fourth child
Charron	Mrs. J. B.	2013	15-Aug-1851	F	fifth child
Chase	Mrs.	777	13-Nov-1842	F	stillborn

33

Obstetrical Casebooks of Dr. F. E. Chatard – an alternative genealogical resource 1829-1883

Chase	Mrs.	1073	13-Nov-1844	M	seventh child
Chase	Mrs. C.	4052	18-Nov-1865	M	fourth pregnancy
Chase	Mrs. Charles	3136	01-Oct-1858	F	second child
Chase	Mrs. Charles	3672	24-Aug-1862	M	third child
Chatard	Mrs.	884	31-Aug-1843	F	sixth child
Chatard	Mrs. Elise	0	25-Mar-1850	F	third child
Chatard	Mrs. Elise	2458	06-Aug-1854	F	fifth child
Chatard	Mrs. F. E.	422	07-Oct-1839	M	fourth child
Chatard	Mrs. F. E.	1654	15-Dec-1848	M	eighth child
Chatard	Mrs. Frederick	1159	26-May-1845	M	first child
Chatard	Mrs. Frederick	1412	28-Mar-1847	F	second child
Chatard	Mrs. Frederick	1830	25-Mar-1850	F	third child
Chatard	Mrs. Frederick	2114	21-Mar-1852	F	fourth child
Chatard	Mrs. Frederick	2850	29-Dec-1856	M	sixth child
Chatard	Mrs. Frederick P.	3307	18-Dec-1859	M	seventh child
Chatard, Jr.	Mrs. F. E.	4987	26-Jun-1875	M	third pregnancy, forceps delivery
Chatard, Jr.	Mrs. F. E.	5209	10-Dec-1879	M	fourth pregnancy
Chatard, Jr.	Mrs. F. E.	5257	18-Aug-1882	F	fifth pregnancy "The child died on the 7th day of cyanosis."
Cheneldine	Mrs. G. N.	3511	25-Apr-1861	F	first child
Chesbrough	Mrs. R.	4228	25-Jun-1867	M	first pregnancy
Chesnut	Mrs. John	5000	28-Aug-1875	F	first pregnancy
Childs	Mrs. Samuel	4638	26-Jan-1871	F	sixth pregnancy
Christel	Mrs. Rosanna	1008	27-Jun-1844	F	labor was completed when I arrived
Christhilf	Mrs. G. H.	718	21-May-1842	M	first child
Christhilf	Mrs. G. H.	878	17-Aug-1843	M	second child

34

Obstetrical Casebooks of Dr. F. E. Chatard – an alternative genealogical resource 1829-1883

Christhilf	Mrs. George	2104	23-Feb-1852	F	seventh child
Christhilf	Mrs. George	2385	22-Jan-1854	M	The child was born before I arrived.
Christhilf	Mrs. George	2708	05-Feb-1856	M/	eighth child, twins
Christhilf	Mrs. George	4290	22-Dec-1867	M	first pregnancy
Christhilf	Mrs. George	4553	26-May-1870	F	second pregnancy
Christie	Mrs. Joseph	4433	25-Mar-1869	M	first pregnancy. ".... made some attempts to breath & cry but soon died."
Christilf	Mrs. G.	1082	03-Dec-1844	M	third child
Christilf	Mrs. George	1327	05-Sep-1846	F	fourth child
Christmer	Mrs. F.	3124	31-Aug-1858	F	third child
Church	Mrs. T. R.	403	04-Aug-1839	F	born 9 PM
Cipriani	Mrs. L.	3345	28-Feb-1860	M	first child. "She was attacked with a severe convulsion. I immediately bled her freely & then delivered her with the forceps. The child proved to be a boy of large size … She died
Clabaugh	Mrs. Usher	5092	13-Nov-1876	M	"The child cried freely after birth and appeared very well but about two hours after birth was attacked with nasal hemorrhage and died about two PM."
Clampitt	Mrs.	407	09-Aug-1839	M	first child
Clark	Mrs.	1091	24-Dec-1844	M	first child, stillborn
Clark	Mrs.	1239	13-Dec-1845	M	second child
Clark	Mrs. J.	1809	04-Feb-1850	M	15th child
Clark	Mrs. James	4889	12-Mar-1874	F	first pregnancy
Clark	Mrs. Joseph	1440	29-May-1847	F	16th child
Clarke	Mrs. Sylvester	3792	16-Jul-1863	F	first pregnancy
Clarke	Mrs. Thomas	1559	07-Apr-1848	M	third child, mother died on 9th or 10th day
Clarke (Rielly)	Mrs.	2118	24-Mar-1852	F	first child
Clelland	Mrs. J.	1710	29-May-1849	F	first child

Obstetrical Casebooks of Dr. F. E. Chatard – an alternative genealogical resource 1829-1883

Clelland	Mrs. J.	2219	12-Dec-1852	M	third child
Clendinen	Mrs. R.	1749	17-Sep-1849	M	born 2:15 AM
Clendinen	Mrs. Thomas R.	5056	21-May-1876	M	first pregnancy
Clendinen	Mrs. Thomas R.	5147	09-Sep-1877	F	second pregnancy
Clendinen	Mrs. Thomas R.	5194	11-Jul-1879	F	third pregnancy
Clendinen	Mrs. Thomas R.	5252	15-Apr-1882	F	fourth pregnancy
Close	Mrs. Alexander	1915	13-Nov-1850	M	first child
Coakley	Mrs. John	2485	23-Sep-1854	F	first child, stillborn
Coakley	Mrs. Michael	3939	29-Oct-1864	F	first pregnancy
Coakley	Mrs. Michael	4196	24-Feb-1867	M	second pregnancy
Coakley	Mrs. Michael	4395	15-Dec-1868	M	third pregnancy
Coale	Mrs. George B.	2961	13-Sep-1857	M	second child
Cobb	Mrs. Josiah	660	28-Nov-1841	M	born 12 PM, died a few hours later
Cobb	Mrs. Josiah	827	03-Mar-1843	M	born 8:30 AM
Cockey	Mrs. C.	4655	27-Apr-1871		eighth pregnancy, seven months, dead
Cockey	Mrs. Covington	2516	28-Nov-1854	M	first child, forceps birth
Cockey	Mrs. Covington	2847	24-Dec-1856	F	second child
Cockey	Mrs. Covington	3181	09-Jan-1859	M	third child
Cockey	Mrs. Covington	3678	10-Sep-1862	M	fourth child
Cockey	Mrs. Covington	4236	26-Jul-1867	M	seventh pregnancy
Cockey	Mrs. Covington	4809	11-Jan-1873	M	ninth pregnancy
Codaghan	Mrs. Edward	2552	01-Feb-1855	M	first child
Codd	Mrs. Edward	3418	12-Sep-1860	F	third child, born dead
Coe	Mrs.	519	21-Aug-1840	M	fourth child
Coe	Mrs. A. B.	789	08-Dec-1842	F	fifth child

36

Surname	Given Name	Number	Date	Sex	Comments
Coe	Mrs. B. A.	1557	28-Mar-1848	F	labor natural & quick the child being born before I arrived
Coen	Mrs.	2642	21-Aug-1855		Nr. 196 Montgomery Street, first child, child died within a few days
Coen	Mrs.	3498	13-Mar-1861	F	
Coffay	Mrs. John	4000	09-May-1865	F	first pregnancy
Coffay	Mrs. Thomas	3448	27-Nov-1860	F	second child
Coffay	Mrs. Thomas	4153	14-Oct-1866	M	fourth pregnancy
Coffay	Mrs. Thomas	4412	30-Jan-1869	F	fifth pregnancy
Coffay	Mrs. Thomas	4756	20-May-1872	F	sixth pregnancy
Cohen	Mrs. E. P.	95	09-Dec-1833	F	second child
Coignet	Mrs. Emile	2266	11-Apr-1853	M	first child
Colardcause	Mrs. F.	3242	27-May-1859	M	second child
Coldtart	Mrs. J.	3246	10-Jun-1859	M	second child
Coldtart	Mrs. John	3458	07-Dec-1860	F	third child
Coldtart	Mrs. John	3681	20-Sep-1862	F	fourth child
Cole	Mrs. Chase	1089	16-Dec-1844	M	first child
Cole	Mrs. J.	742	03-Aug-1842	M	first child
Cole	Mrs. J. R.	03-Jun-1840	miscarriage at four weeks		

Page 59

Surname	Given Name	Number	Date	Sex	Comments
Cole	Mrs. J. R.	745	16-Aug-1842	M	
Cole	Mrs. John R.	376	05-Apr-1839	M	third child

Obstetrical Casebooks of Dr. F. E. Chatard – an alternative genealogical resource 1829-1883

Surname	Given Name	Number	Date	Sex	Comments
Cole	Mrs. John R.	1043	16-Sep-1844	F	sixth child
Cole	Mrs. John R.	1333	13-Sep-1846	F	sixth child
Cole	Mrs. John R.	2135	23-May-1852	F	eighth child
Cole	Mrs. W. A.	921	21-Nov-1843	M	second child
Cole	Mrs. W. A.	1128	14-Feb-1845	F	third child
Cole	Mrs. W. A.	1364	06-Dec-1846	F	fourth child
Cole	Mrs. W. A.	1800	25-Jan-1850	F	fifth child
Cole	Mrs. W. A.	2010	09-Aug-1851	F	sixth child
Cole	Mrs. W. A.	2238	09-Feb-1853	F	seventh child
Cole	Mrs. W. R.	2700	11-Jan-1856	F	first child
Cole	Mrs. W. R.	4820	07-Mar-1873	M	eighth pregnancy
Cole	Mrs. William R.	3456	06-Dec-1860	F	third child
Cole	Mrs. Wm.	4204	28-Mar-1867	M	sixth pregnancy

Page 60

Surname	Given Name	Number	Date	Sex	Comments
Cole	Mrs. Wm.	4446	08-May-1869	F	seventh pregnancy
Cole	Mrs. Wm. A.	3733	14-Jan-1863	F	fourth child
Cole	Mrs. Wm. R.	3114	20-Aug-1858	F	second child
Cole, Jr.	Mrs. Isaac	4506	30-Nov-1869	F	first pregnancy
Coleman	Mrs. Frederic W.	5088	02-Nov-1876	F	first pregnancy
Collier	Mrs. C.	4508	04-Dec-1869	M	sixth pregnancy
Collier	Mrs. Charles	2992	06-Nov-1857	M	first child
Collier	Mrs. Charles	3296	19-Nov-1859	M	second child

Obstetrical Casebooks of Dr. F. E. Chatard – an alternative genealogical resource 1829-1883

Collier	Mrs. Charles	3600	19-Dec-1861	M	third child
Collier	Mrs. Charles	3966	31-Dec-1864	F	fourth pregnancy. "The mother had variola whilst in her 7th month of gestation. The child was healthy & presented no marks of the disease."
Collier	Mrs. Henry	3193	03-Feb-1859	F	second child
Collier	Mrs. Henry	3438	02-Nov-1860	M	fourth child
Collier	Mrs. Henry	3660	21-Jul-1862	M	fifth child
Collinean	Mrs. L. G.	2662	29-Sep-1855	M	first child
Collins	Mrs.	1571	29-Apr-1848	F	second child
Collins	Mrs.	1803	26-Jan-1850	F	first child
Collins	Mrs. J.	3427	09-Oct-1860	M	first child
Collins	Mrs. Mary	3014	03-Dec-1857	at St. Vincent's Asylum, first child	
Coltart	Mrs. John	3026	27-Dec-1857	F	first child
Colter	Mrs. John	4935	19-Sep-1874	F	second pregnancy
Colton	Mrs. John	2514	23-Nov-1854	M	first child
Colton	Mrs. John	2900	11-May-1857	F	second child
Colton	Mrs. John	4811	18-Jan-1873		first pregnancy
Colton	Mrs. John	5165	15-Aug-1878	M	fourth pregnancy
Coltor	Mrs. John	5031	08-Jan-1876	M	third pregnancy
Conally	Mrs. John	233	05-May-1837	F	born about 1/2 hour after I arrived

Obstetrical Casebooks of Dr. F. E. Chatard – an alternative genealogical resource 1829-1883

Conally	Mrs. John	378	07-Apr-1839		three months miscarriage
Conklin	Elizabeth	2017	22-Aug-1851	M	colored, seventh child, stillborn
Conklin	Mrs. William	2783	15-Aug-1856	M	colored. Second child
Conncell	Mrs. J. F.	3729	03-Jan-1863	M	fourth child
Connelly	Mrs. M.	11-Feb-1841			three month miscarriage
Connelly	Mrs. Michael	1003	18-Jun-1844	F	born 9:30 AM
Connelly	Mrs. Richard	1671	08-Feb-1849	M	fifth child
Connlly	Mrs. M.	446	30-Dec-1839	M	fourth child
Connolly	Mrs.	768	20-Oct-1842	M	first child
Connelly	Mrs. Hugh	3633	02-May-1862	M	second child
Connelly	Mrs. M.	724	14-Jun-1842	M	13th child, stillborn
Connelly	Mrs. M.	843	02-May-1843	M	eighth child
Connolly	Mrs. Michael	23-Jun-1841			miscarriage at three months
Connolly	Mrs. Michael	1834	16-Apr-1850	M	13th child
Connolly	Mrs. Patrick	2614	05-Jul-1855	F	nr. 105 Harford Avenue, 11th child
Connolly	Mrs. R.	26-Jul-1847	M		fourth child, attended by Dr Benke
Connolly	Mrs. R.	1005	20-Jun-1844	F	second child
Connolly	Mrs. R.	1269	28-Mar-1846	F	third child, attended by Dr Diffenderfer
Connolly	Mrs. Richard	1878	22-Aug-1850	M	seventh child
Connolly	Mrs. Richard	2216	08-Dec-1852	F	seventh child

40

Obstetrical Casebooks of Dr. F. E. Chatard – an alternative genealogical resource 1829-1883

Connoly	Mrs. Hugh	3489	10-Feb-1861	F	first child
Connor	Mrs. F.	4924	18-Aug-1874		second pregnancy
Connor	Mrs. Francis	3642	27-May-1862	F	ninth child
Connor	Mrs. Frank	4790	28-Oct-1872	M	first pregnancy
Connor	Mrs. Thomas	4691	24-Sep-1871	F	first pregnancy
Conroy	Mrs. I.	4339	11-Jan-1868	F	fifth pregnancy
Conroy	Mrs. J.	4191	16-Feb-1867	F	fourth pregnancy
Conroy	Mrs. John	2627	06-Aug-1855	F/F	first child, twins, second dead
Conroy	Mrs. John	3535	18-Jun-1861	M	third child
Constable	Mrs.	2996	11-Nov-1857	F	fourth child
Contee	Mrs. Benjamin	2982	15-Oct-1857	M	first child, stillborn
Cook	Mrs. Frank	3018	18-Dec-1857	F	first child
Cook	Mrs. Frank	3567	09-Sep-1861	F	second child
Cook	Mrs. S. G. B.	4874	31-Dec-1873	F	third pregnancy
Cook	Mrs. Saml. G. B.	4384	10-Nov-1868		first pregnancy, seven months, "did not survive more than a couple of days."
Cook	Mrs. Saml. G. B.	4504	17-Nov-1869	M	second pregnancy
Cook	Mrs. W. G. B.	5044	10-Mar-1876	F	fourth pregnancy
Coolaghan	Mrs. John	3801	10-Aug-1863	F	first pregnancy, patient of Dr J. O'Donovan. Child dead. "The patient remained very feeble & died about an hour after."
Coonan	Mrs. Michael J.	4068	31-Dec-1865	F	second pregnancy
Cooney	Mrs. W. G. T.	4165	08-Dec-1866	F	first pregnancy
Cooper	Mrs.	94	29-Dec-1833	M	first child
Cooper	Mrs. Wm.	1205	19-Sep-1845	F	second child

Obstetrical Casebooks of Dr. F. E. Chatard – an alternative genealogical resource 1829-1883

Cooran	Mrs. Michael	3832	28-Dec-1863	M	first child
Corner	Mrs. George	1138	30-Mar-1845	M	first child
Corrigan	Mrs. John	2244	21-Feb-1853	F	second child
Corrigan	Mrs. John	2427	22-May-1854	M	third child
Corrigan	Mrs. John	2728	25-Mar-1856	F	fourth child. "All her previous labors had terminated in the death of the child."
Corrigan	Mrs. John	3130	10-Sep-1858	M	fifth child
Cosgrove	Mrs. Patrick	2906	26-May-1857	F	fifth child
Coskery	Mrs. Dr. Oscar J.	5071	31-Jul-1876	M	first pregnancy, forceps delivery
Coss	Mrs. George	186	27-Apr-1836	F	first child
Coss	Mrs. George	252	06-Sep-1837	F	second child, eighth month
Coss	Mrs. George	353	03-Dec-1838	M	third child
Coss	Mrs. George	452	07-Jan-1840	M	fourth child
Coss	Mrs. George	587	21-Apr-1841	M	fifth child
Coss	Mrs. George	872	30-Jul-1843	F	sixth child
Coss	Mrs. George	1354	12-Nov-1846	M	
Costaggini	Mrs. Phillip	4841	26-Jun-1873	F	first pregnancy
Costaggini	Mrs. Phillip	4982	05-Jun-1875	M	second pregnancy
Costaggini	Mrs. Phillip	5087	26-Oct-1876	F	third pregnancy
Cotter	Mrs. John	3394	18-Jul-1860	M	first child
Cottman	Mrs.	1104	18-Jan-1845	M	first child
Coulson	Mrs.	1429	02-May-1847	F	first child
Coulter	Mrs.	261	03-Oct-1837	M	
Coulter	Mrs. James M	3453	02-Dec-1860	F	second child

Obstetrical Casebooks of Dr. F. E. Chatard – an alternative genealogical resource 1829-1883

Coulter	Mrs. James M.	3896	13-Jun-1864	M	fourth pregnancy
Coulter	Mrs. James M.	3087	26-May-1858	M	first child
Coulter	Mrs. James M.	3734	14-Jan-1863	F	third child
Coulter	Mrs. James M.	3896	13-Jun-1864	M	fourth pregnancy
Coulter	Mrs. James M.	4194	20-Feb-1867	M	fifth pregnancy
Coulter	Mrs. James M.	4396	22-Dec-1863	F	sixth pregnancy
Coulter	Mrs. John	3592	17-Nov-1861	F	fourth child
Coulton	Mrs. John	3255	13-Jul-1859	M	third child
Councell	Mrs. J. F.	3073	14-Apr-1858	F	third child
Counsell	Mrs. J. F.	2747	12-May-1856	M	second child
Courcelle	Mrs. Adrien	4414	03-Feb-1869	M	third pregnancy
Courtois	Mrs. Armand	869	23-Jul-1843	M	third child
Cox	Mrs. James G.	920	19-Nov-1843	F	second child
Cox	Mrs. James G.	1219	22-Oct-1845	F	third child. She was attacked with puerperal fever and died on the 5th November
Coyne	Mrs. Mary	1663	17-Jan-1849	M	first child
Craig	Mrs. C. B.	2228	12-Jan-1853	F	fourth child
Crane	Mrs. A. P.	4320	02-Apr-1868	M	second pregnancy
Crane	Mrs. A. P.	4939	01-Oct-1874	F	fourth pregnancy
Crane	Mrs. James C.	5093	22-Nov-1876	F	first pregnancy
Cranford	Mrs. Margaret	3196	07-Feb-1859	F	at St. Vincent's Asylum, first child
Crawford	Mrs.	93	27-Dec-1833	F	eighth child. Previous children were all boys
Crawford	Mrs.	172	25-Dec-1835	F	first child
Crawford	Mrs.	184	22-Apr-1836	F	resided at Franklin St., fifth child
Crawford	Mrs.	263	05-Oct-1837	M	second child
Crawford	Mrs. B. A.	443	16-Dec-1839	F	third child

43

Obstetrical Casebooks of Dr. F. E. Chatard – an alternative genealogical resource 1829-1883

Crawford	Mrs. B. A.	804	04-Jan-1843	M	fourth child
Crawford	Mrs. John L.	4234	12-Jul-1867	F	first pregnancy
Crawford	Mrs. John L.	4531	08-Mar-1870	M	second pregnancy
Crawford	Mrs. W. H.	3806	20-Aug-1863	F	second child
Crawford	Mrs. W. H.	4034	25-Sep-1865		third pregnancy. "The child gave no signs of life having died from internal hemorrhage."
Crawford	Mrs. W. H.	4214	01-May-1867	F	fourth pregnancy, eighth month, child dead
Crawford	Mrs. W. H.	4670	16-Jun-1871	F	sixth month, child stillborn
Crawford	Mrs. William	4750	27-Apr-1872	M	"I found her very pale and pulse weak & complaining of being faint on

44

Obstetrical Casebooks of Dr. F. E. Chatard – an alternative genealogical resource 1829-1883

Crawford	Mrs. Wm.	3676	02-Sep-1862	M	rising," stillborn
Crawford	Mrs. Wm. H.	4353	17-Jul-1868	M	first child, forceps delivery, stillborn
Cremer	Mrs. S. A.	5234	13-Mar-188	M	fifth pregnancy
Cremer	Mrs. S. A.	5253	19-Apr-1882	F	third pregnancy
Cremer	Mrs. Stephen A.	5129	20-Jun-1877	M	fourth pregnancy
Cremer	Mrs. Stephen A.	5204	19-Oct-1879	F	first pregnancy
Crengels	Mrs. John	414	04-Sep-1839	M	second pregnancy
Crengles	Mrs.	51	16-Aug-1832	M	seventh child
Crengles	Mrs.	109	17-Jun-1834	F	see 7 Sep 1831 [#27]. Third child.
Crengles	Mrs.	185	27-Apr-1836	F	see 15 Aug 1832 [#51], fourth child
Crengles	Mrs.	1690	19-Mar-1849	F	see 17 Jun 1834 [#109], fifth child
Crengles	Mrs. John	277	05-Jan-1838	F	13th child
Crengles	Mrs. John	600	03-Jun-1841	F	sixth child
Crengles	Mrs. John	972	21-Mar-1844	M	born 3:15 PM
Crimmons	Mrs. T.	3941	04-Nov-1864	M	born about 10:30 PM
Crimmons	Mrs. Timothy	3396	19-Jul-1860	M	sixth pregnancy
Crinmous [?]	Mrs.	2575	30-Mar-1855	M	fourth child
Crise	Mrs. J. L.	650	27-Oct-184	M	first child
Crise	Mrs. J. L.	932	10-Dec-1843	F	first child
Crise	Mrs. J. L.	1337	22-Sep-1846	F	second child
Crise	Mrs. J. L.	1919	24-Nov-1850	M	third child
Crise	Mrs. J. L.	2310	26-Jul-1853	M	stillborn
Crise	Mrs. J. L.	2628	06-Aug-1855	M	sixth child
Crise	Mrs. John L.	1649	28-Nov-1848	F	seventh child
Cromwell	Mrs. Mary	3626	18-Apr-1862	M	fourth child
					first child

45

Obstetrical Casebooks of Dr. F. E. Chatard – an alternative genealogical resource 1829-1883

Cromwell	Mrs. Richard	3866	15-Mar-1864	M	second pregnancy
Cromwell	Mrs. Richard	4101	11-May-1866	F	third pregnancy
Cromwell	Mrs. Richard	4326	18-Apr-1868	M	fourth pregnancy
Cromwell	Mrs. Richard	4576	24-Jul-1870	F	fifth pregnancy
Cromwell	Mrs. Richard	4686	05-Aug-1871	M	sixth pregnancy
Cronglet	Mrs. John	27	07-Sep-1831	M	aged 23. Six months. "There was some appearance of labor attended with great cerebral derangement. The head was shaved & mustard applied." Child died
Crook	Mrs. Francis	460	10-Feb-1840	F	first child
Crook	Mrs. Henry	2199	05-Nov-1852	F	first child
Crook	Mrs. Joseph	816	30-Jan-1843	M	seventh child
Crook	Mrs. Joseph	986	28-Apr-1844	F	tenth child
Crook	Mrs. Walter	716	09-May-1842	M	second child
Cross	Mrs.	2586	24-Apr-1855		first child, dead
Crouch	Mrs. M. T.	4261	03-Oct-1867	M	first pregnancy
Crown	Mrs. J. R.	4501	09-Nov-1869	F	third pregnancy, "All her previous labours had been very difficult & long."
Crown	Mrs. J. R.	4675	07-Jul-1871	F	fourth pregnancy, "She insisted upon taking chloroform, which arrested the uterine contractions. I then at her earnest request applied the forceps."
Crummins	Mrs.	2746	07-May-1856	M	third child
Cruter	Mrs.	122	03-Nov-1834	M	first child
Cugle, Jr.	Mrs. John	3767	08-Apr-1863	M	first pregnancy
Cullen	Mrs. James	3216	22-Mar-1859	F	fourth child
Cullen	Mrs. James	3412	30-Aug-1860	M	fifth child
Culter	Mrs. Charles	2329	07-Sep-1853	M	second child

46

Obstetrical Casebooks of Dr. F. E. Chatard – an alternative genealogical resource 1829-1883

Culter	Mrs. Charles	3127	04-Sep-1858	M	fifth child
Cummings	Mrs. W. A.	3799	08-Aug-1863	M	first pregnancy
Cunningham	Mrs.	614	29-Jul-1841	M	first child
Cunningham	Mrs. James	626	18-Aug-1841	M	first child
Cunningham	Mrs. James	909	26-Oct-1843	F	second child
Cunningham	Mrs. William	5178	22-Jan-1879	F	second pregnancy
Curley	Mrs.	214	04-Nov-1836	M	third child
Curley	Mrs. Bernard	2739	22-Apr-1856	M	second child
Curley	Mrs. Bernard	3023	21-Dec-1857	M	third child
Curley	Mrs. H.	355	10-Dec-1838	F	fourth child
Curley	Mrs. Henry	505	29-Jun-1840	F	fifth child
Curley	Mrs. Henry	761	15-Sep-1842	M	sixth child
Curley	Mrs. J. W.	723	06-Jun-1842	M	sixth child
Curley	Mrs. James	265	06-Oct-1837	M	third child
Curley	Mrs. James	369	04-Mar-1839	F	fourth child
Curley	Mrs. James W.	551	28-Nov-1840	F	fifth child
Curley	Mrs. James W.	987	29-Apr-1844	F	seventh child
Curley	Mrs. James W.	1257	02-Feb-1846	F	eighth child
Curley	Mrs. James W.	1479	16-Sep-1847	M	ninth child
Curley	Mrs. James W.	1754	28-Sep-1849	F	tenth child
Curley	Mrs. James W.	2041	19-Oct-1851	F	11th child
Curran	Mrs.	866	12-Jul-1843	M	first child
Curtis	Catherine	3128	05-Sep-1858	M	colored, attended by Drs Milkellan & VanBibber, child dead
Curtis	Mrs. J. A.	4249	01-Sep-1867	F	third pregnancy
Cushing	Mrs.	654	08-Nov-1841	M	fourth child
Cushing	Mrs. David	2392	07-Feb-1854	F	ninth child

47

Obstetrical Casebooks of Dr. F. E. Chatard – an alternative genealogical resource 1829-1883

Cushing	Mrs. George	1185	02-Aug-1845	F	fourth child
Cushing	Mrs. George	1448	26-Jun-1847	M	fifth child
Cushing died	Mrs. George	1600	10-Jul-1848	M	nearly 40 years of age, first child, mother
Cushman	Mrs. Cephas	2926	25-Jun-1857	F	second child
Cutler	Mrs. Charles	2057	12-Nov-1851	M	first child
Cutler	Mrs. Charles	2640	19-Aug-1855	F	third child
Cutler	Mrs. Charles	2846	21-Dec-1856	F	fourth child
Cutler	Mrs. Charles	3624	03-Apr-1862	F	seventh child
Cutler	Mrs. Charles	3907	17-Jul-1864	M	eighth pregnancy
Cutter	Mrs. Charles	3428	11-Oct-1860	F	sixth child
Dailey	Mrs. E.	3745	15-Feb-1863	M	first pregnancy
Dailey	Mrs. Eugene	3977	22-Jan-1865	M	second pregnancy
Dallam	Mrs. John	743	04-Aug-1842	M	first child
Dallam	Mrs. John	1050	12-Oct-1844	M	second child
Dallam	Mrs. John	2360	28-Nov-1853	M	fourth child
D'Almaine	Mrs.	1396	14-Feb-1847	F	second child
Dalton	Mrs. James	2142	31-May-1852	F	first child
Daly	Mrs. E.	4992	30-Jul-1875	M	seventh pregnancy
Daly	Mrs. Eugene	4149	08-Oct-1866	M	third pregnancy
Daly	Mrs. Eugene	4299	27-Jan-1868	M	fourth pregnancy
Daly	Mrs. Eugene	4438	13-Apr-1869	M	fifth pregnancy
Daly	Mrs. Eugene	4747	25-Apr-1872	M	sixth pregnancy
Damman	Mrs.	1007	26-Jun-1844	M	second child
Damman	Mrs. F. W.	1506	30-Nov-1847	M	fourth child

Obstetrical Casebooks of Dr. F. E. Chatard – an alternative genealogical resource 1829-1883

Damman	Mrs. Francis	4765	09-Jul-1872	F	first pregnancy
Damman	Mrs. J. F.	4967	05-Jan-1875	F	second pregnancy
Damman	Mrs. J. F>	5106	23-Feb-1877	F	third pregnancy
Damman	Mrs. W. F.	1846	24-May-1850	F	born 9:45 PM
Damman	Mrs. W. F.	2284	21-May-1853	M/	twins
Damman	Mrs. W. F.	2530	21-Dec-1854	F	11th child
Damman	Mrs. W. F.	2801	05-Oct-1856	M	11th child
Damman	Mrs. Wm. F.	1685	07-Mar-1849	F	deformed child died at 36 hours
Dandelet	Mrs.	1562	17-Apr-1848	M	first child
Dandelet	Mrs. F.	1941	30-Jan-1851	M	third child
Dandelet	Mrs. F.	3126	02-Sep-1858	M	second child
Dandelet	Mrs. F.	3770	13-Apr-1863	M	third pregnancy
Dandelet	Mrs. Francis	2599	25-May-1855	M	first child
Dandelet	Mrs. Francis	3297	21-Nov-1859	F	(Hammond), sixth child
Dandelet	Mrs. Francois	4015	19-Jun-1865	F	fourth pregnancy
Dandelet	Mrs. Lucile	2230	15-Jan-1853	F	fourth child
Daniel	Mrs. J. H.	2078	23-Dec-1851	F	sixth child
Danman	Mrs. Ernest	2923	23-Jun-1857	M	first child, forceps delivery
Danman	Mrs. J. F.	5221	26-Jul-1880	M	fifth pregnancy
Danman	Mrs. John F.	5172	24-Oct-1878	F	fourth pregnancy
Danmar	Mrs. F. W.	2116	22-Mar-1852	F	seventh child
Dannenberg	Mrs. F. K.	1117	06-Feb-1845	F	third child
Dannenberg	Mrs. F. K.	1361	02-Dec-1846	F	fourth child
Darrell	Mrs. S.	4923	16-Aug-1874	F	second pregnancy
Darrell	Mrs. Stewart	4805	16-Dec-1872	M	first pregnancy
D'Arville	Mrs. Edward	4195	21-Feb-1867	M	first pregnancy

Obstetrical Casebooks of Dr. F. E. Chatard – an alternative genealogical resource 1829-1883

Davies	Mrs. Richard	489	11-May-1840	M	first child
Davis	Mrs. C. J.	2083	15-Jan-1852	M	second child
Dawson	Mrs. W. P.	3926	21-Sep-1864	M	second pregnancy. "I applied the forceps & extracted the child … Six years before she was delivered by me in the same manner."
Dawson	Mrs. William	3145	13-Oct-1858	F	first child
De Katow	Mrs. A.	4730	06-Jan-1872	F	first pregnancy
de Les Sarter	Mrs. S.	3160	06-Nov-1858	F	second child
Deanery	Mrs. J.	3829	13-Dec-1863	M	first child
Deannery	Mrs. J.	3983	05-Feb-1865	M	second pregnancy
Deaver	Mrs. George	4365	19-Aug-1868	F	colored, second pregnancy
Deaver	Mrs. George	5146	02-Sep-1877	M	colored, sixth pregnancy
Deavitt	Mrs. Elizabeth	2717	02-Mar-1856	M	second child
Debering	Mrs. G.	1636	21-Oct-1848	M	third child
Debering	Mrs. J. G.	3005	18-Nov-1857	F	ninth child
deBonneville	Mrs.	1167	16-Jun-1845	F	second child
Debring	Mrs.	1313	05-Aug-1846	F	third child
Debring	Mrs. G.	2591	09-May-1855	M	seventh child
Debring	Mrs. G.	2770	19-Jul-1856	M	eighth child
Debring	Mrs. J. G.	1908	03-Nov-1850	F	fifth child
Debring	Mrs. J. G.	2234	25-Jan-1853	F	sixth child
Deck	Mrs. John	1860	05-Jul-1850	F	first child, forceps, difficult delivery
Deckar [Drohar]	Mrs. Thomas	1674	14-Feb-1849		born 5 PM
Decker	Mrs. C.	1469	18-Aug-1847		third child, five months, child died
Decker	Mrs. C.	1585	06-Jun-1848	F	fourth child
Decker	Mrs. C.	1945	08-Feb-1851	F	Fifth child

50

Obstetrical Casebooks of Dr. F. E. Chatard – an alternative genealogical resource 1829-1883

Dedier	Mrs. Eugene	4957	30-Nov-1874	F	first pregnancy, "three weeks short of her full period."
Deecke	Mrs. G. C.	1198	29-Aug-1845	F	second child
DeFord	Mrs. George	3115	22-Aug-1858	F	third child
DeFord	Mrs. W. T.	3481	25-Jan-1861	M	fourth child
deFord	Mrs. W. Y.	2127	22-Apr-1852	F	first child
deFord	Mrs. W. Y.	2313	31-Jul-1853	M	second child
deFord	Mrs. Wm.	2727	17-Mar-1856	F	third child
Deihl	Mrs. John	4238	07-Aug-1867	M	first pregnancy
Deihl	Mrs. Louisa	4402	01-Jan-1869	M	second pregnancy
Deiter	Mrs. V.	1968	05-Apr-1851	M	fourth child
Deitrich	Mrs. Charles	4559	15-Jun-1870	F	second pregnancy
DeKatow	Mrs. A.	4849	03-Aug-1873	F	third pregnancy
DeKatow	Mrs. A.	4985	11-Jun-1875	F	fourth pregnancy
DeKatow	Mrs. A.	5126	11-Jun-1877	F	fifth pregnancy
Delaney	Mrs.	821	18-Feb-1843	M	first child
Delaney	Mrs.	1060	20-Oct-1844	F	second child
Delaney	Mrs. Charles	1535	28-Jan-1848	F	third child
Delaney	Mrs. Charles	1922	29-Nov-1850	M	fourth child
Delaney	Mrs. Charles	2263	05-Apr-1853	F	fifth child
Delaney	Mrs. Charles	2782	14-Aug-1855	F	sixth child
Delker	Mrs. John C.	615	30-Jul-1841	M	second child, stillborn
Dell	Mrs. George E.	5065	07-Jul-1876	F	first pregnancy
Dellam	Mrs. J.	2006	28-Jul-1851	F	third child
Delmas	Mrs. Alexis	57	04-Nov-1832	F	first child, eight months, four pounds. "Both mother & child did well."
Denison	Mrs. J. M.	4086	26-Feb-1866	M	premature at 5.5 months
Denison	Mrs. John M.	5241	24-Aug-1881	M	second pregnancy

51

Obstetrical Casebooks of Dr. F. E. Chatard – an alternative genealogical resource 1829-1883

Denison	Mrs. Robert M.	3994	22-Apr-1865	F	second pregnancy
Denmead, Jr.	Mrs. Edward	2879	13-Mar-1857	F	first child
Dennis	Mrs. J. U.	3908	20-Jul-1864	M	first pregnancy. "It must have been dead six weeks or two months."
Dennis	Mrs. James U.	4038	06-Oct-1865	M	second pregnancy
Dennison	Mrs. Robert	4108	19-Jun-1866	M	third pregnancy
Denny	Mrs. W. A.	4081	13-Feb-1866	F	first pregnancy
Derouges	Madame	1001	12-Jun-1844	M	fourth child
deSantes	Mrs. Mary	2842	13-Dec-1856	M	first child
deSouza	Mrs. Lally	5196	16-Jul-1879	M	first pregnancy
Devaux	Madame P.	927	02-Dec-1843	M	third child
Devaux	Mrs.	283	20-Feb-1838	M/F	fourth child. Twins one male, one female
Devaux	Mrs.	431	06-Nov-1839	M	fourth child
Devaux	Mrs. John	938	30-Dec-1843	M	fourth child
Devaux	Mrs. John	1253	27-Jan-1846	F	fifth child
Devonge	Madame	1728	21-Jul-1849	F	sixth child
Devonges	Mrs. A.	1426	30-Apr-1847	F	fifth child
Devonges	Mrs. A.	4622	13-Dec-1870	M	first pregnancy
Devonges	Mrs. A.	5116	18-Apr-1877	M	fourth pregnancy, child dead
Devonges	Mrs. A.	5260	11-Oct-1882	M	sixth pregnancy
Devonges	Mrs. Alphonse	4952	10-Nov-1874	F	second pregnancy
Devonges	Mrs. Alphonse	5052	23-Apr-1876	M	third pregnancy
Devonges	Mrs. Alphonse	5214	07-Feb-1880	M	fifth pregnancy
Dickinson	Mrs. Henry E.	2097	06-Feb-1852	M	first child
Didier	Mrs. Eugene	5218	15-May-1880	F	case, gave her a dose of Bromide of Potash."
Didier	Mrs. Henry	4406	12-Jan-1869	M	third pregnancy
Didier	Mrs. John	2954	28-Aug-1857	M	first child

52

Obstetrical Casebooks of Dr. F. E. Chatard – an alternative genealogical resource 1829-1883

Diffenderffer	D'Arcy Mrs. Michael	4538	21-Apr-1870	F	first pregnancy
Diggs	Mrs. J. R.	4846	20-Jul-1873	M	first pregnancy
Dignan	Mrs. Peter	3755	07-Mar-1863	M	first pregnancy
Dignan	Mrs. Peter	4170	24-Dec-1866	F	third pregnancy
Dise	Mrs. J. T.	2398	24-Feb-1854	F	first child
Dobbin	Mrs. G. W.	992	09-May-1844	M	sixth child
Dobbin	Mrs. Thomas M.	5032	12-Jan-1876	F	first pregnancy, forceps delivery
Dobbins	Mrs. J. T.	3909	21-Jul-1864	M	second pregnancy
Dodge	Mrs.	1168	18-Jun-1845	M	third child
Doffay	Mrs. Thomas	3759	11-Mar-1863	M	third child
Doize	Mrs. Henry	1096	31-Dec-1844	F	born 3:30 PM
Doize	Mrs. Henry	1933	08-Jan-1851	F	11th child
Doize	Mrs. Henry	2253	13-Mar-1853	F	12th child
Doizé	Mrs. Henry	1394	10-Feb-1847	M	ninth child
Doizé	Mrs. Henry	1691	19-Mar-1849	F	tenth child
Doizet	Mrs.	174	30-Dec-1835	M	see 5 Dec 1834 [#127], third child
Doizet	Mrs.	234	11-May-1837	M	fourth child
Doizet	Mrs.	815	29-Jan-1843	F	seventh child
Dolan	Mrs.	18	07-Aug-1830	first child	
Dolan	Mrs.	47	18-Jul-1832	F	see 7 Aug 1830 [#18]; second child
Dolan	Mrs. Martin	1980	30-May-1851	M	first child
Donaghe	Mrs. Dr. Briscoe	4082	01-Feb-1866	F	fourth pregnancy

53

Obstetrical Casebooks of Dr. F. E. Chatard – an alternative genealogical resource 1829-1883

Donahue	Mrs. Cornelius	2577	02-Apr-1855	M	11th child
Donahue	Mrs. Cornelius	2818	27-Oct-1856	F	tenth child
Donaldson	Mrs. Thomas	409	01-Aug-1839	F	first child, 10 pounds
Donn	Mrs.	4115	12-Jul-1866	F	first pregnancy
Donn	Mrs. John W.	4300	29-Jan-1868	F	second pregnancy
Donnally	Mrs.	453	07-Jan-1840		miscarriage at four months
Donnally	Mrs.	561	27-Dec-1840	M	first child
Donnell	Mrs. J. M.	3769	12-Apr-1863	M	seventh pregnancy
Donnell	Mrs. William	3303	12-Dec-1859	F	first child
Donnelly	Mrs. D.	3063	29-Mar-1858	F	second child
Donnelly	Mrs. Daniel	2836	06-Dec-1856	F	first child
Donnelly	Mrs. Daniel	3436	29-Oct-1860	M	third child
Donnelly	Mrs. Daniel	3725	29-Dec-1862	M	fourth child
Donnelly	Mrs. Daniel	3967	31-Dec-1864	F	fifth pregnancy
Donovan	Mrs.	1371	27-Dec-1846	M	sixth child
Donovan	Mrs. Timothy	1814	14-Feb-1850	F	seventh child, died slightly after birth
Dooley	Mrs. Delia	4783	27-Sep-1872	M	first pregnancy, "aged about 40 years, a very long & tedious labour." child died
Dorget	Mrs. H.	577	25-Feb-1841	F	sixth child
Dorman	Mrs. John	478	07-Apr-1840	M	first child, still born, difficult birth
Dorman	Mrs. John	593	01-May-1841	F	second child. Infant died next day
Dorman	Mrs. John	886	05-Sep-1843	F	stillborn
Dorsey	Mrs. Bartus C.	4649	09-Apr-1871	M	first pregnancy
Dorsey	Mrs. Catherine	1312	02-Aug-1846	F	fifth child
Dorsey	Mrs. Catherine	1569	26-Apr-1848	F	sixth child, stillborn

54

Obstetrical Casebooks of Dr. F. E. Chatard – an alternative genealogical resource 1829-1883

Dorsey	Mrs. Catherine	2221	15-Dec-1852	M	ninth child
Dorsey	Mrs. E. G.	3930	26-Sep-1864	M	fifth pregnancy
Dorsey	Mrs. E. H.	204	17-Sep-1836	M	fifth child
Dorsey	Mrs. Lorenzo	314	19-Jul-1838	M	first child
Dorsey	Mrs. Lorenzo	537	24-Oct-1840	F	second child
Dorsey	Mrs. W. H.	1746	11-Sep-1849	M	seventh child
Dorsey	Mrs. W. H. G.	2978	10-Oct-1857	F	third child
Dorsey	Mrs. W. H. G.	2502	23-Oct-1854	M	fifth child
Dorsey	Mrs. W. R.	2056	11-Nov-1851	F	eighth child, stillborn
Dorsey	Mrs. Wm. H. G.	2804	07-Oct-1856	F	second child
Dorsey	Mrs. Wm. R.	2609	26-Jun-1855	M	tenth child
D'Orville	Mrs. A.	1252	24-Jan-1846	F	born 6 AM
Dougherty	Mrs. James	524	19-Sep-1840	F	11th child
Dougherty	Mrs. James	704	07-Apr-1842	F	12th child
Dougherty	Mrs. James	1187	03-Aug-1845	M	14th child, died a few minutes after birth
Dougherty	Mrs. James	1320	20-Aug-1846	M	15th child
Dougherty	Mrs. James	1525	11-Jan-1848	M	16th child
Dougherty	Mrs. Susan	2753	22-May-1856	M	at St. Vincent's Asylum, first child
Doughterty	Mrs. James	1721	04-Jul-1849	M	17th child
Douglass	Mrs. August	4789	26-Oct-1872	M	fifth pregnancy
Douglass	Mrs. Joseph	1094	30-Dec-1844	F	
Douglass	Mrs. Joseph	1529	16-Jan-1848	M	sixth child
Douglass	Mrs. Joseph	1934	10-Jan-1851	M	seventh child
Douglass	Mrs. Soloman	4132	11-Aug-1865	M	colored, first pregnancy
Downing	Mrs. H.	375	03-Apr-1839	F	second child

Obstetrical Casebooks of Dr. F. E. Chatard – an alternative genealogical resource 1829-1883

Doyle	Mrs.	1340	24-Sep-1846		first child, stillborn
Doyle	Mrs.	1478	14-Sep-1847	M	second child
Doyle	Mrs. Charles J.	5212	14-Jan-1880	F	third pregnancy
Doyle	Mrs. Edward	3747	19-Feb-1863	M	fourth pregnancy
Doyle	Mrs. James	2311	30-Jul-1853	M	first child
Doyle	Mrs. Michael	2606	12-Jun-1855	F	third child
Doyle	Mrs. Michael	2742	27-Apr-1856	M	attended by Dr McSherry, child dead. Mother died 28th
Doyle	Mrs. Michael	4103	19-May-1866	M	first pregnancy
Doyle	Mrs. Michael	4329	04-May-1868	M	second pregnancy
Doyle	Mrs. Patrick	3553	11-Aug-1861	M	first child, stillborn
Doyle	Mrs. Patrick	3651	27-Jun-1862	M	second child
Doyle	Mrs. Patrick	3890	20-May-1864	F	third pregnancy
Doyle	Mrs. Patrick	4045	30-Oct-1865	M	fourth pregnancy
Doyle	Mrs. Peter	1637	27-Oct-1848	M	seventh child
Doyle	Mrs. Peter	2012	14-Aug-1851	F/F	twins, premature 6 months
Doyle	Mrs. Peter	2272	27-Apr-1853	F	born 3:45 PM
Doyle	Mrs. Peter	4502	14-Nov-1869	M	(Decker St.) fourth pregnancy
Doyle	Mrs. Peter	4694	30-Sep-1871	F	Duker St., fifth pregnancy
Doyle	Mrs. Peter	4872	26-Dec-1873	F	sixth pregnancy
Doyle	Mrs. Peter	4994	03-Aug-1875	M	seventh pregnancy
Doyle	Mrs. Thomas	2191	17-Oct-1852	M	first child
Doyle	Mrs. Thomas	2367	15-Dec-1853	F	second child
Doyle	Mrs. Thomas	2744	02-May-1856	M	third child
Doyle	Mrs. Thomas	3022	19-Dec-1857	M	fourth child
Doyle	Mrs. Thomas	3295	18-Nov-1859	M	fourth child. "It lived but a short time."

Obstetrical Casebooks of Dr. F. E. Chatard – an alternative genealogical resource 1829-1883

Doyle	Mrs. Thomas	3484	31-Jan-1861	F	fifth child
Doyle	Mrs. Thomas	3630	23-Apr-1862	F	seventh child
Doyle	Mrs. Thomas	3920	30-Aug-1864	F	eighth pregnancy
Doyle	Mrs. Thomas	4138	22-Aug-1866	M	ninth pregnancy
Doyle	Mrs. Thomas	4354	22-Jul-1868	M	tenth pregnancy
Doyle	Mrs. Thomas	4662	13-May-1871	M	11th pregnancy
Doyle	Mrs. Thomas	4882	26-Jan-1874	M	12th pregnancy
Doyle	Mrs. Thomas	4989	04-Jul-1875	F	13th pregnancy
Doyle	Mrs. William	3225	25-Apr-1859	M	eighth child
Doyle	Mrs. William	3657	14-Jul-1862	F	tenth child
Doyle	Mrs. Wm.	2105	25-Feb-1852	F	fourth child
Doyle	Mrs. Wm.	2355	17-Nov-1853	F	fifth child
Doyle	Mrs. Wm.	2681	21-Nov-1855	M	sixth child. "It died a few minutes after birth."
Doyle	Mrs. Wm.	2832	27-Nov-1856	M	seventh child
Doyle	Mrs. Wm.	3544	20-Jul-1861	F	ninth child
Doyle	Mrs. Wm.	4344	23-Jun-1868	M	12th pregnancy
Draghar	Mrs. Thomas	2466	18-Aug-1854	F	14th child
Drain	Mrs. Richard	3372	21-May-1860	M	first child
Drane	Mrs. Richard	3609	23-Jan-1862	F	second child
Drew	Mrs. Arthur	4111	29-Jun-1866	M	second pregnancy
Drizet	Mrs.	127	05-Dec-1834	M	second child, nine pounds
Drohan	Mrs. Thomas	1191	14-Aug-1845	M	ninth child
Drohan	Mrs. Thomas	1880	30-Aug-1850	M	12th child
Dryden	Mrs. C. O.	4817	24-Feb-1873	F	first pregnancy
Dryden	Mrs. C. O.	4915	17-Jul-1874	F	second pregnancy
Dryden	Mrs. J. R.	3275	25-Sep-1859	M	seventh child

57

Obstetrical Casebooks of Dr. F. E. Chatard – an alternative genealogical resource 1829-1883

Dryden	Mrs. Joshua	1218	20-Oct-1845	F	first child
Dryden	Mrs. Joshua	1684	06-Mar-1849	M	fifth child
Dryden	Mrs. Joshua	1863	20-Jul-1850	M	fourth child
Dryden	Mrs. Joshua R.	2112	13-Mar-1852	M	sixth child
Dryden	Mrs. Joshua R.	3000	14-Nov-1857	F	sixth child
Dryden, Jr.	Mrs. Joshua	1455	25-Jul-1847	F	second child
Dubarry	Mrs. Ernest	4516	21-Dec-1869	F	first pregnancy
Dubois	Mrs.	433	07-Nov-1839	M	
Dubois	Mrs. E.	344	29-Oct-1838	F	a colored woman, second child
Dubois	Mrs. Emile	557	08-Dec-1840	M	colored, fourth child
Dubois	Mrs. Joseph	227	18-Mar-1837	F	first child
Dubois	Mrs. Joseph	731	29-Jun-1842	M	colored, five months, child died
Duer	Mrs.	1362	05-Dec-1846	M	first child
Duering	Mrs. George S.	4907	11-Jun-1874	F	first pregnancy
Duffy	Mrs. Hugh	386	26-May-1839	F	second child
Duffy	Mrs. Hugh	960	11-Feb-1844	M	fourth child
Dugan	Mrs. C.	3698	01-Nov-1862	F	sixth child
Dugan	Mrs. Cumberland	2922	22-Jun-1857	F	first child
Dugan	Mrs. Cumberland	3104	27-Jul-1858	M	second child
Dugan	Mrs. Cumberland	3269	08-Sep-1859	M	third child
Dugan	Mrs. Cumberland	3402	02-Aug-1860	M	fourth child

58

Obstetrical Casebooks of Dr. F. E. Chatard – an alternative genealogical resource 1829-1883

Dugan	Mrs. Cumberland	3570	18-Sep-1861	M	fifth child
Dugan	Mrs. Cumberland	3873	30-Mar-1864	M	seventh pregnancy
Dugan	Mrs. Cumberland	4012	06-Jun-1865	F	eighth pregnancy
Dugan	Mrs. Cumberland	4136	19-Aug-1866	F	ninth pregnancy
Dugan	Mrs. Cumberland	4276	07-Nov-1867	F/F	tenth pregnancy
Dugan	Mrs. Cumberland	4424	01-Mar-1869	M	11th pregnancy
Dugan	Mrs. Cumberland	4581	01-Aug-1870	M	12th pregnancy
Dugan	Mrs. Cumberland	4740	17-Mar-1872	M	13th pregnancy
Dugan	Mrs. Hammond	4227	17-Jun-1867	M	first pregnancy
Dulaney	Mrs. G. L.	612	27-Jul-1841	M	fifth child
Dulaney	Mrs. G. L.	1121	11-Feb-1845	F	sixth child
Dulaney	Mrs. J. M.	4706	20-Nov-1871	M	first pregnancy
Dulany	Mrs. J. M.	5107	11-Mar-1877	F	fourth pregnancy
Dulany	Mrs. John	4845	07-Jul-1873	M	second pregnancy
Dumbleton	Mrs. J. A.	1617	19-Sep-1848	M	third child
Dunbar	Mrs. George	798	22-Dec-1842	M	third child
Duncan	Mrs.	1496	26-Oct-1847	M	of HocksTown Road, attended by Dr Buckler, stillborn
Duncan	Mrs. Edward	3693	26-Oct-1862	F	sixth child

Obstetrical Casebooks of Dr. F. E. Chatard – an alternative genealogical resource 1829-1883

Dunkin	Mrs. Levi	2040	18-Oct-1851	M	11th child
Dunlap	Mrs. A.	4945	29-Oct-1874	F	fourth pregnancy
Dunlap	Mrs. A.	5173	11-Nov-1878	M	sixth pregnancy
Dunlap	Mrs. A. H.	4278	13-Nov-1867	M	second pregnancy
Dunlap	Mrs. A. H.	4758	06-Jun-1872	M	third pregnancy
Dunlap	Mrs. Amasa H.	5139	25-Jul-1877	F	fifth pregnancy
Dunlap	Mrs. Charles	1739	03-Sep-1849	M	fourth child
Dunlap	Mrs. Charles	3086	24-May-1858	F	fifth child. "Nine years had elapsed since the birth of her previous child."
Dunlap	Mrs. Charles	3454	02-Dec-1860	M	first child
Dunn	Mrs.	808	09-Jan-1843	M	ninth child, died within hours
Dunn	Mrs. Michael	2123	18-Apr-1852	F	tenth child, stillborn
Dunn	Mrs. Michael	4572	14-Jul-1870	F	fifth pregnancy
Durand	Mrs. Rosalie	2432	31-May-1854	M	second child
Durce	Mrs.	447	01-Jan-1840	M	colored woman attended by midwife
Dushane	Mrs. A. J.	3944	15-Nov-1864	F	second pregnancy
Dushane	Mrs. J. A.	3278	03-Oct-1859	F	first child
Dusquesne	Madame	1866	30-Jul-1850	F	second child
Dutch	Mrs.	202	11-Sep-1836	F	first child
Dutch	Mrs.	309	06-Jul-1838	F	second child
Dutch	Mrs.	658	26-Nov-1841	F	fourth child, severe hemorrhage
Dutch	Mrs. M.	449	03-Jan-1840	F	third child
Dutch	Mrs. W. N.	930	09-Dec-1843	M	fifth child
Dutch	Mrs. W. N.	1270	01-Apr-1846	F	sixth child
Duvall	Mrs.	544	22-Nov-1840	F	

Obstetrical Casebooks of Dr. F. E. Chatard – an alternative genealogical resource 1829-1883

Duvall	Mrs. Charles	4239	09-Aug-1867	M	first pregnancy
Duvall	Mrs. Charles	4634	16-Jan-1871	M	second pregnancy
Duvall	Mrs. Eldridge	1896	05-Oct-1850	F	fifth child
Duvall	Mrs. L. C.	1242	24-Dec-1845	F	third child. She became deranged from over excitement and died on the 19th day.
Duvall	Mrs. Langdon C.	784	29-Nov-1842	M	born 4 PM
Duvall	Mrs. Langdon C.	1034	02-Sep-1844	M	second child, child born before I arrived
Duvall	Mrs. Richard	1108	25-Jan-1845	F	born 10:30 PM
Dver	Mrs. P. S.	3446	24-Nov-1860	M	fifth child
Dydenhoover	Mrs. W.	1711	02-Jun-1849	M	first child
Dyer	Mrs. J. Baker	4371	06-Sep-1868	M	first pregnancy
E.	Mrs.	538	29-Oct-1840	F	seventh child
Earl	Mrs.	895	25-Sep-1843	M	third child
Early	Mrs. Samuel	2792	16-Sep-1856	M	first child
Easter	Mrs. J.	2607	13-Jun-1855	M	third child
Easter	Mrs. James H.	2202	09-Nov-1852	M	second child
Easter	Mrs. James H.	2848	26-Dec-1856	M	fourth child
Easter	Mrs. James H.	3804	16-Aug-1863	M	first pregnancy
Easter	Mrs. James H.	3949	27-Nov-1864	M	second pregnancy
Easter	Mrs. W. S.	4940	02-Oct-1847,	F	first pregnancy
Eaton	Mrs. George	3015	08-Dec-1857	F	sixth child
Edgar	Mrs. H.	946	18-Jan-1844	F	third child
Edmonds	Mrs. Samuel	3910	21-Jul-1864	F	first pregnancy
Edwards	Mrs.	1994	27-Jun-1851	M	first child

61

Obstetrical Casebooks of Dr. F. E. Chatard – an alternative genealogical resource 1829-1883

Edwards	Mrs. Edward J.	4033	23-Sep-1865		first pregnancy
Edwards	Mrs. George W.	5222	10-Sep-1880	M	first pregnancy
Edwards	Mrs. J. E.	5004	14-Sep-1875	F	fourth pregnancy
Edwards	Mrs. J. R>	5206	19-Sep-1879	M	fifth pregnancy
Edwards	Mrs. R.	2761	16-Jun-1856	F	third child
Edwards	Mrs. R.	3144	10-Oct-1858	F	fourth child
Edwards, Jr.	Mrs. Richard	484	25-Apr-1840	M	third child
Egerton	Mrs. A. D.	2307	19-Jul-1853	M	first child
Egbert	Mrs. Dr.	1735	31-Jul-1849	F	fifth child
Egerton	Mrs. A. D.	2511	13-Nov-1854	F	second child
Egerton	Mrs. A. D.	3384	21-Jun-1860	F	third child
Egerton	Mrs. C. C.	758	10-Sep-1842	F	second child
Egerton	Mrs. C. C.	1057	18-Oct-1844	F	third child
Egerton	Mrs. C. C.	1334	18-Sep-1846	M	fourth child
Egerton	Mrs. C. C.	1628	08-Oct-1848	F	fifth child
Egerton	Mrs. C. C.	1901	16-Oct-1850	F	sixth child
Egerton	Mrs. C. C.	2227	10-Jan-1853	M	sixth child
Egerton	Mrs. C.C.	546	23-Nov-1840	F	first child
Egerton	Mrs. J. C.	4582	29-Aug-1870	F	first pregnancy
Egerton, Jr.	Mrs. C. C.	2596	14-May-1855	M	seventh child
Ehler	Mrs.	1602	22-Jul-1848	M	first child
Eichelberger	Mrs.	699	29-Mar-1842	M	third child
Eichelberger	Mrs. William	3332	26-Jan-1860	F	second child
Eichenberger	Mrs. Phillip	2778	05-Aug-1856	M	first child
Eichman	Mrs. C.	4264	20-Oct-1867	M	second pregnancy

62

Obstetrical Casebooks of Dr. F. E. Chatard – an alternative genealogical resource 1829-1883

Eichman	Mrs. J. C.	5109	16-Mar-1877	F	sixth pregnancy
Eichner	Mrs. C.	4884	04-Feb-1874	M	fifth pregnancy
Elder	Mrs. Basil T.	1589	25-Jun-1848	F	born half past 12 AM
Elder	Mrs. Basil T.	1859	04-Jul-1850	F	born 11 AM
Elder	Mrs. Basil T.	2091	25-Jan-1852	M	eighth child
Elder	Mrs. Basil T.	2358	27-Nov-1853	F	ninth child
Elder	Mrs. Basil T.	2678	14-Nov-1855	M	tenth child
Elder	Mrs. Francis	1596	01-Jul-1848	F	born 4:30 PM
Elder	Mrs. Francis	3222	20-Apr-1859	F	first child
Elder	Mrs. Francis	4200	04-Mar-1867	M	second pregnancy
Elder	Mrs. Robert	3712	05-Dec-1862	F	first child
Elder	Mrs. Robert	3913	28-Jul-1864	F	second pregnancy
Elder	Mrs. Robert	4206	08-Apr-1867	M	third pregnancy
Eldridge	Mrs. R. B.	3033	09-Jan-1858	F	fourth child
Ellett	Mrs. F. M.	4231	29-Jun-1867	M	first pregnancy
Ellett	Mrs. F. M.	4383	10-Nov-1868	F	second pregnancy
Ellett	Mrs. F. M.	4652	16-Apr-1871	F	third pregnancy
Ellicott	Mrs.	599	02-Jun-1841	F	third child
Ellicott	Mrs.	1085	06-Dec-1844	M	fourth child
Ellicott	Mrs. Edward	1020	10-Aug-1844	F	second child
Ellicott	Mrs. Edward T	1432	15-May-1847	M	third child
Ellis	Mrs. Henry	491	14-May-1840	M	fifth child
Elmer	Mrs. W. F.	4786	12-Oct-1872	F	first pregnancy
Emcy	Mrs. Richard	3083	15-May-1858	M	fourth child
Emery	Mrs. Daniel	2774	27-Jul-1856	F	first child
Emmans [?]	Mrs. Dr.	1349	01-Nov-1846	F	second child, delivered by Dr. Bailey

63

Obstetrical Casebooks of Dr. F. E. Chatard – an alternative genealogical resource 1829-1883

Emmins	Mrs. George	3330	24-Jan-1860	M	sixth child
Emmons	Mrs. George	2144	06-Jun-1852	M	fourth child
Emmons	Mrs. George	2944	31-Jul-1857	M	fifth child
Emmons	Mrs. Lt.	1907	02-Nov-1850	M	third child
Emory	Mrs.	900	07-Oct-1843	F	fifth child
Emory	Mrs. D. C. H.	1406	24-Mar-1847	M	seventh child
Emory	Mrs. D. C. H.	2247	22-Feb-1853	M	10th child
Emory	Mrs. Daniel	3150	20-Oct-1858	F	second child. Mother developed pneumonia and died on the 24th.
Emory	Mrs. Hopper	1076	21-Nov-1844	F	
Emory	Mrs. W.	1468	17-Aug-1847	M	fourth child
Emory	Mrs. W. J.	1190	11-Aug-1845	F	fourth child
English	Mrs. J.	3998	03-May-1865	M	second pregnancy
English	Mrs. John	3726	31-Dec-1862	F	first child, attended by Dr. D. McKen
English	Mrs. John	4213	26-Apr-1867	M	third pregnancy
Ensey	Mrs. R. F.	2595	14-May-1855	M	third child
Ensey	Mrs. Richard	2420	07-May-1854	F	second child
Ensey	Mrs. Richard	3430	19-Oct-1860	M	fifth child
Ensey	Mrs. Richard	3655	09-Jul-1862	M	sixth child
Ensey	Mrs. Richard	4087	28-Feb-1866	M	seventh pregnancy
Ensey	Mrs. Richard	4243	24-Aug-1867	M	eighth pregnancy
Esmery	Mrs. Alfred J. B.	5025	18-Dec-1875	F	first pregnancy, six months, child died after a few hours
Essert	Mrs.	363	09-Feb-1839	M	third child
Eton	Mrs. Benjamin	1835	19-Apr-1850	F	first child
Eustis	Mrs. A. B.	3206	08-Mar-1859	F	seventh child

Obstetrical Casebooks of Dr. F. E. Chatard – an alternative genealogical resource 1829–1883

Evans	Mrs.	1563	18-Apr-1848	M	first child, he died in a few days
Evans	Mrs. George	3692	22-Oct-1862	M	first child
Evans	Mrs. George	4281	16-Nov-1867	M	third pregnancy
Evans	Mrs. Henry	3752	27-Feb-1863	M	second pregnancy
Evans	Mrs. Henry	3887	10-May-1864	F	third pregnancy
Evans	Mrs. Henry	4155	28-Oct-1866	F	fourth pregnancy
Evans	Mrs. Henry C.	3582	07-Nov-1861	M	first child
Everhardt	Mrs. William	3437	01-Nov-1860	F	first child
Everhart	Mrs. Martin	1974	07-May-1851	M	second child
Fagan	Mrs. Owen	1176	10-Jul-1845	M	second child
Fagret	Madame	2380	14-Jan-1854	F	second child
Fagret	Mrs.	1888	12-Sep-1850	M	first child
Fagret	Mrs. F	2821	09-Nov-1856	F	third child
Fahey	Mrs. James	2634	14-Aug-1855	M	first child
Fahey	Mrs. Patrick	2883	20-Mar-1857	M	first child
Fahey	Mrs. Thomas	2646	02-Sep-1855	M	second child. "The child showed no signs of life."
Fahey	Mrs. Thomas	2812	21-Oct-1856	M	third child
Fahey	Mrs. Thomas	3194	05-Feb-1859	M	fourth child, died. Mother died 10 AM 6 Feb 1859. " ... Did not appear to suffer much."
Fahey	Mrs. Thomas	4023	29-Aug-1865	F	first pregnancy
Fair	Mrs. Campbell	5007	03-Oct-1875	F	first pregnancy, "excessive anasarca." child dead
Fairbanks	Mrs. William	3375	26-May-1860	M	first child, attended by Dr. J. Thomas. Forceps delivery
Fairfield	Mrs. S. L.	317	23-Jul-1838	M	sixth child
Falconar	Mrs. John	1892	25-Sep-1850	F	third child
Fallon	Mrs. John	3	03-Sep-1829		22 years old, first child; "The child was troubled by cholera which was removed by a little sweet oil and tepid water."

65

Obstetrical Casebooks of Dr. F. E. Chatard – an alternative genealogical resource 1829-1883

Fallon	Mrs. Malachai	4169	24-Dec-1866	M	first pregnancy
Fallon	Mrs. Rebecca	2910	05-Jun-1857	F	first child
Falls	Mrs. M.	949	20-Jan-1844	F	sixth child
Falls [Falks]	Mrs. Morris N.	1395	12-Feb-1847	F	seventh child
Farnac	Mrs. J.	4687	10-Aug-1871	M	second pregnancy
Farran	Mrs. James	4524	18-Jan-1870	M	first pregnancy, "The child a large boy with a very firmly ossified head was stillborn giving no sign of life."
Farrell	Mrs. James	2545	21-Jan-1855	F	first child. "The child when born made a few attempts to breath but soon died."
Farrell	Mrs. James	2692	18-Dec-1855	M	second child
Farrell	Mrs. Matthew	5048	03-Apr-1876	F	first pregnancy
Farris	Mrs. J. E>	3986	02-Mar-1865	M	first pregnancy. ". . . taken with a severe pain in her head in the evening of the 25th, about one AM she was attacked with convulsions."
Faucit	Mrs. Len [?]	1704	26-Apr-1849	F	first child
Fay	Mrs. James	2975	08-Oct-1857	M	first child
Fay	Mrs. James	3359	14-Apr-1860	M	second child
Feast	Mrs. John	903	13-Oct-1843	F	sixth child
Fedan	Mrs.	1542	18-Feb-1848	F/F	first child, twins
Fedon	Mrs.	1937	14-Jan-1851	F	second child
Fedon	Mrs.	2390	04-Feb-1854	M	third child
Fegan	Mrs.	41	16-Jan-1832	F	first child
Fegan	Mrs.	1553	19-Mar-1848	F	born 8 AM
Fegan	Mrs.	2115	22-Mar-1852	M	first child
Fegan	Mrs. Owen	1829	22-Mar-1850	F	fourth child
Fegan	Mrs. Owen	2243	21-Feb-1853	F	fifth child
Fegan	Mrs. Owen	2682	22-Nov-1855	M	fifth child

Obstetrical Casebooks of Dr. F. E. Chatard – an alternative genealogical resource 1829-1883

Fegan	Mrs. Owen	3209	15-Mar-1859	F	seventh child
Fegan	Mrs. Peter	2468	26-Aug-1854	M	second child
Fegan	Mrs. Peter	2759	09-Jun-1856	M	third child
Felton	Mrs. James	2504	25-Oct-1854	M	first child
Fickey	Mrs. F.	343	20-Oct-1838	M	ninth child
Fields	Mrs.	171	24-Dec-1835	F	first child
Fillinger	Mrs.	302	18-May-1838	F	first child
Fillinger	Mrs. P.	450	05-Jan-1840	F	second child
Fillinger	Mrs. Paul	715	08-May-1842	M	third child
Fimple	Mrs.	641	12-Oct-1841	F	first child
Finaughty	Mrs. John	2550	26-Jan-1855	M	first child
Findlay	Mrs. J. V. L.	4071	10-Jan-1866	M	second pregnancy
Findlay	Mrs. J. V. L.	4280	14-Nov-1867	F	third pregnancy
Finlay	Mrs.	17	23-Jul-1830		fourth or fifth child, child died of icterus on 8th or 9th day
Finlay	Mrs.	3877	09-Apr-1864	M	first pregnancy, daughter of Dr J. O. Mackenzie & attended by her brother Dr J. C. Mackenzie
Finlay	Mrs. James	1534	27-Jan-1848	F	first child
Finlay	Mrs. James	1763	17-Oct-1849	F	second child
Finlay	Mrs. James	1936	13-Jan-1851	F	third child
Finlay	Mrs. James J.	2129	26-Apr-1852	M	fourth child
Finlay	Mrs. James J.	2361	02-Dec-1853	F	fifth child
Finlay	Mrs. James J.	2593	12-May-1855	M	sixth child
Finlay	Mrs. James J.	2809	17-Oct-1856	F	seventh child
Finlay	Mrs. John	4178	23-Jan-1867	F	second pregnancy
Finlay	Mrs. John F.	2005	18-Jul-1851	F	first child

67

Obstetrical Casebooks of Dr. F. E. Chatard – an alternative genealogical resource 1829-1883

Finlay	Mrs. John J.	2523	08-Dec-1854	F	second child
Finlay	Mrs. John J.	2833	28-Nov-1856	F	third child
Finley	Mrs. James	3224	25-Apr-1859	F	ninth child
Finley	Mrs. James J.	3071	11-Apr-1858	M	eighth child
Finley	Mrs. James J.	3364	11-May-1860	F	tenth child
Finley	Mrs. James J.	3628	21-Apr-1862	F	11th child
Finley	Mrs. James J.	3975	21-Jan-1865	F	13th pregnancy
Finley	Mrs. John	3178	24-Dec-1858	M	fourth child
Finley	Mrs. John	4394	11-Dec-1868	F	third pregnancy
Finley	Mrs. John F.	4785	03-Oct-1872	F	fifth pregnancy
Finley	Mrs. John J.	3973	15-Jan-1865	F	first pregnancy
Finley	Mrs. John S.	3455	04-Dec-1860	M	premature labor, fifth child, lived but a short time
Finn	Mrs. D.	3981	03-Feb-1865	F	second pregnancy
Finnard	Mrs.	2070	11-Dec-1851	F	second child
Fischer	Mrs. George	300	26-Apr-1838	mother & child died	
Fisher	Mrs.	1483	23-Sep-1847	M	second child
Fisher	Mrs. G. W.	1815	15-Feb-1850	M	third child
Fisher	Mrs. G. W.	2168	25-Aug-1852	F	fourth child, attended by Dr. Knight
Fisher	Mrs. G. W.	2571	20-Mar-1855	M	seventh child
Fisher	Mrs. G. W.	2990	25-Oct-1857	F	sixth child
Fisher	Mrs. G. W.	3325	13-Jan-1860	M	seventh child
Fisher	Mrs. G. W.	3936	12-Oct-1864	F	ninth pregnancy
Fisher	Mrs. J. J.	1575	11-May-1848	F	7 months, brought on prematurely by her little daughter, who fell on

Obstetrical Casebooks of Dr. F. E. Chatard – an alternative genealogical resource 1829-1883

Fisher	Mrs. N. D.	4588	15-Sep-1870	M	mother's abdomen
Fisher	Mrs. Richard D.	3815	10-Oct-1863	F	fourth pregnancy
Fisher	Mrs. Richard D.	4049	14-Nov-1865	F	first pregnancy
Fisher	Mrs. Richard D.	4327	24-Apr-1868	M	second pregnancy
Fisher	Mrs. Richard D.	4996	07-Aug-1875	M	third pregnancy
Fisher	Mrs. S.	3791	12-Jul-1863	M	sixth pregnancy
Fiskey	Mrs.	655	14-Nov-184-	M	fifth pregnancy
Fitzberger	Mrs. H.	2080	31-Dec-1851	F	born 9:30 PM
Fitzpatric	Mrs. J. J.	158	09-Sep-1835	F	fifth child
Fitzpatrick	Mrs.	2297	20-Jun-1853	F	first child
Fitzpatrick	Mrs. Mary	3286	27-Oct-1859	F	first child
Fitzpatrick	Mrs. Wm.	2851	12-Jan-1857	M	at St. Vincent's Asylum, eighth child
Fitzsimmons	Mrs. Christopher	3722	22-Dec-1862	M	first child
Fitzsimmons	Mrs. Daniel	2696	31-Dec-1855	M	third child
Flack	Mrs. G. W.	937	28-Dec-1843	M	fourth child. "Called to her accidentally"
Flack	Mrs. G. W.	1254	31-Jan-1846	M	third child
Flaherty	Mrs. C.	2303	09-Jul-1853	M	fourth child
Flaherty	Mrs. C.	2546	21-Jan-1855	F	second child
Flaherty	Mrs. Patrick	2064	01-Dec-1851	M	third child
Flaherty	Mrs. Pierce	3451	01-Dec-1860	F	first child
Flannigan	Mrs. I.	4521	02-Jan-1870	M	second child, stillborn, forceps delivery
Flannigan	Mrs. J.	4883	31-Jan-1874	F	second pregnancy
Flannigan	Mrs. James	4367	29-Aug-1868	M	third pregnancy
Fledderman	Mrs. H. G.	3479	20-Jan-1861	M	first pregnancy, "The child showed no signs of life."
					first child

69

Obstetrical Casebooks of Dr. F. E. Chatard – an alternative genealogical resource 1829-1883

Flemming	Mrs. Thomas	2185	30-Sep-1852	M	second child
Flemming	Mrs. Thomas	2643	24-Aug-1855	F	second child
Flemming	Mrs. Thomas	3149	19-Oct-1858	F	third child
Flintlock	Mrs. E.	1415	02-Apr-1847	F	first child
Flintsbeck	Mrs.	1957	02-Mar-1851	M	second child, mother died on 18th day
Floyd	Mrs.	143	19-Apr-1835	F	tenth child
Flynn	Mrs.	167	23-Nov-1835	M	first child
Flynn	Mrs. Patrick	3187	22-Jan-1859	M	fifth child
Foard	Mrs. A. K.	2572	20-Mar-1855	M	third child
Foard	Mrs. A. K.	2903	19-May-1857	M	fourth child
Foard	Mrs. Addison K.	2348	02-Nov-1853	M	second child
Fondriak	Mrs.	1414	02-Apr-1847	F	born about 6 AM
Force	Mrs.	259	20-Sep-1837	M	third child, 9.5 pounds
Ford	Ann	1093	29-Dec-1844	F	colored
Ford	Mrs. E. J.	2373	03-Jan-1854	F	second child
Ford	Mrs. Edward	1876	11-Aug-1850	F	first child
Ford	Mrs. J. G.	1997	10-Jul-1851	F	first child
Ford	Mrs. Wm.	2426	21-May-1854	M	third child
Forley	Mrs. Patrick	2178	11-Sep-1852	F	first child
Forley	Mrs. Patrick	2375	07-Jan-1854	F	second child
Forno	Mrs.	193	14-Jul-1836	M	first child
Forrest	Mrs.	1595	01-Jul-1848	M	first child
Forsyth	Mrs. D.	3574	28-Sep-1861	M	third child
Forsyth	Mrs. David	2964	18-Sep-1857	M	first child
Forsyth	Mrs. David	3292	14-Nov-1859	F	second child

Obstetrical Casebooks of Dr. F. E. Chatard – an alternative genealogical resource 1829-1883

Fort	Mrs. Allen I.	4026	04-Sep-1865	F	third pregnancy
Fortune	Mrs.	79	29-Jul-1833	F	"Feeble constitution."
Fortune	Mrs.	155	29-Jul-1835	F	see 29 Jul 1833 [#79], seven months, third child
Fortune	Mrs.	242	03-Aug-1837	M	fourth child, died 36 hours later
Fortune	Mrs.	310	08-Jul-1838	F	fourth child
Fortune	Mrs. James	575	11-Feb-184_	M	born 1:30 AM
Foster	Mrs. J. W.	3317	07-Jan-1860	M	third child
Foster	Mrs. James W.	4250	03-Sep-1867	M	third pregnancy
Foussé	Mrs. F.	4257	20-Sep-1867		first pregnancy
Fowler	Mrs. E. C.	3285	26-Oct-1859	F	first child
Fowler	Mrs. E. C.	3507	14-Apr-1861	F	second child
Fowler	Mrs. E. C.	3691	20-Oct-1862	M	third child
Fowler	Mrs. E. C.	4027	05-Sep-1865		fifth pregnancy
Fowler	Mrs. J. P.	4032	22-Sep-1865	F	first pregnancy
Fowler	Mrs. J. P.	4390	24-Nov-1868	F	second pregnancy
Fowler	Mrs. W.	1173	05-Jul-1845	F	first child
Fowler	Mrs. W.	1348	28-Oct-1846	M	second child
Fowler	Mrs. W. H.	1686	07-Mar-1849	F	third child
Fox	Mrs. J. T.	4533	22-Mar-1870	F	first pregnancy, forceps delivery
Fox	Mrs. James	2663	02-Oct-1855	M	first child
Fox	Mrs. Tazewell	4749	27-Apr-1872	F	third pregnancy
Fox	Mrs. W. Tazewell	4653	19-Apr-1871	M	second pregnancy
Fox	Mrs. W. Tazewell	4887	24-Feb-1874	F	fourth pregnancy

Obstetrical Casebooks of Dr. F. E. Chatard – an alternative genealogical resource 1829-1883

Fox	Mrs. W. Tazewell	5064	02-Jul-1876	M	fifth pregnancy
Foy	Mrs. J. H.	3748	19-Feb-1863	F	second pregnancy
Foy	Mrs. J. H.	4226	16-Jun-1867	M	fourth pregnancy
Foy	Mrs. J. Henry	3556	18-Aug-1861	F	first child
Foy	Mrs. J.H.	3957	12-Dec-1864	M	third pregnancy
Frailey	Mrs. George C.	1694	25-Mar-1849	F	fourth child
Frailey	Mrs. George	1927	19-Dec-1850	M	fifth child
France	Mrs. Joseph	2068	08-Dec-1851	M	fifth child
France	Mrs. William	4331	06-May-1868	M	fifth pregnancy
France	Mrs. Wm.	3002	15-Nov-1857	M	second child
Francis	Mrs. James	3962	24-Dec-1864	M	second pregnancy
Frazier	Mrs. Edward	1646	17-Nov-1848	F	first child
Fredericks	Mrs. J. M.	2007	01-Aug-1851	F	fifth child
Freiderich	Mrs. J. Ph.	2386	27-Jan-1854	F	sixth child
French	Mrs. Joseph	969	15-Mar-1844	F	first child
French	Mrs. Joseph	1221	03-Nov-1845	M	second child
French	Mrs. Joseph	1477	12-Sep-1847	M	third child
French	Mrs. Joseph	1841	09-May-1850	F	fifth child
Frizelle	Mrs. John	3717	18-Dec-1862	M	first child
Fuller	Mrs.	947	19-Jan-1844	F	second child
Gaietey	Mrs. Patrick	3635	10-May-1862	F	first child, forceps delivery
Gaiety	Mrs. P.	3857	13-Feb-1864	F	second pregnancy
Gaiety	Mrs. Patrick	4186	05-Feb-1867	F	third pregnancy
Gaiety	Mrs. Patrick	4392	03-Dec-1868	F	fourth pregnancy
Gale	Mrs. Samuel	3096	18-Jun-1858	M	first child

Obstetrical Casebooks of Dr. F. E. Chatard – an alternative genealogical resource 1829-1883

Surname	Given	#	Date	Sex	Notes
Gale	Mrs. Susan	2844	19-Dec-1856	F	first child
Gallagher	Mrs.	215	08-Nov-1836	M	miscarriage of five months
Gallagher	Mrs.	1996	06-Jul-1851	M	third child, complicated birth
Gallagher	Mrs. E.	2312	30-Jul-1853	M	second child
Gallagher	Mrs. Edward	2953	25-Aug-1857	M	third child
Gallagher	Mrs. Edward	3786	18-Jun-1863	M	fifth pregnancy
Gallagher	Mrs. Francis	3590	16-Nov-1861	M	second child
Gallagher	Mrs. Francis	3803	15-Aug-1863	M	third pregnancy
Gallagher	Mrs. Francis	4886	19-Feb-1874	F	fifth pregnancy
Gallagher	Mrs. Francis	5024	17-Dec-1875		sixth pregnancy
Gallagher	Mrs. Francis J.	3349	09-Mar-1860	F	first child
Gallagher	Mrs. James	2814	24-Oct-1856		first child
Gallagher	Mrs. James	3038	28-Jan-1858	F	second child
Gallagher	Mrs. James	3223	21-Apr-1859	M	third child
Gallagher	Mrs. James	3465	16-Dec-1860	F	fourth child
Gallagher	Mrs. James	3810	31-Aug-1863	F	sixth pregnancy
Gallagher	Mrs. James	3991	11-Apr-1865	F	seventh pregnancy
Gallagher	Mrs. Joseph	3874	02-Apr-1864	M	first pregnancy
Gallagher	Mrs. Joseph	4089	02-Mar-1866	M	second pregnancy
Gallagher	Mrs. Joseph	4335	21-May-1868	M	third pregnancy
Gallagher	Mrs. Patrick	2334	18-Sep-1853	M	at 14 West Fayette St, first child
Gallagher	Mrs. Patrick	2557	16-Feb-1855	M	born 12:30 PM
Gallagher	Mrs. Philip	2704	26-Jan-1856	M	first child, stillborn
Gallagher	Mrs. William	5077	18-Aug-1876	M	third pregnancy
Gallegher	Mrs. Phillip	2861	14-Feb-1857	M	second child

Obstetrical Casebooks of Dr. F. E. Chatard – an alternative genealogical resource 1829-1883

Galvin	Mrs. Patrick	4401	31-Dec-1868	M	third pregnancy
Galvin	Mrs. Wm.	3917	06-Aug-1864	M	first pregnancy
Gambrill	Mrs. B. F.	4917	23-Jul-1874	M	first pregnancy
Ganory [?]	Mrs. F. X.	4808	23-Dec-1872	M	second pregnancy
Gardiner	Mrs. Lewis	4797	24-Nov-1872	M	first pregnancy
Gardiner	Mrs. Louis	4899	20-Apr-1874	M	second pregnancy
Gardiner	Mrs. Louis	5210	11-Dec-1879	M	fourth pregnancy
Gardner	Mrs.	254	08-Sep-1837	M	first child
Gardner	Mrs.	461	11-Feb-1840	M	second child
Gardner	Mrs. J. M.	3043	14-Feb-1858	M	second child, died shortly after birth
Garnett	Mrs. Dr.	4251	06-Sep-1867	M	third pregnancy
Garrett	Mrs. J. C.	1960	07-Mar-1851	M	third child
Garrett	Mrs. J. Harrison	4608	14-Nov-1870	F	first pregnancy
Garrett	Mrs. J. Harrison	4848	01-Aug-1873	M	third pregnancy
Garrett	Mrs. J. Harrison	4986	24-Jun-1875	M	fourth pregnancy
Garrett	Mrs. J. Harrison	5160	14-Jun-1878	F	fifth pregnancy, the child was dead. "Her recovery was favorable."
Garrett	Mrs. J. W.	1420	09-Apr-1847	M	first child
Garrett	Mrs. J. W.	1672	11-Feb-1849	M	second child
Garrett	Mrs. John C.	2400	08-Mar-1854	F	fourth child
Garrett	Mrs. T. Harrison	4755	19-May-1872	M	second pregnancy
Garry	Mrs. B.	2205	15-Nov-1852	F	first child
Garvey	Mrs. J.	4210	23-Apr-1867	F	first pregnancy
Garvey	Mrs. James	4611	19-Nov-1870	F	fourth pregnancy
Garvey	Mrs. Michael	3207	10-Mar-1859	M	first child
Gassaway	Mrs. Henry	3955	09-Dec-1864	F	first pregnancy

74

Obstetrical Casebooks of Dr. F. E. Chatard – an alternative genealogical resource 1829-1883

Gassaway	Mrs. Henry	4411	25-Jan-1869	M	third pregnancy
Gatchell	Mrs.	136	04-Feb-1835	M	fifth child, ten pounds
Gatchell	Mrs.	225	18-Feb-1837	M	sixth child
Gatchell	Mrs.	389	03-Jun-1839	F	seventh child
Gatchell	Mrs. W.	677	19-Jan-1842	M	born 11 AM
Gatchell	Mrs. Wm.	1051	14-Oct-1844	M	fourth [or ninth] child
Gatt delivery	Mrs.	210	06-Oct-1836	F	second child, attended by midwife, forceps
Gault	Mrs. Cyrus	854	13-Jun-1843	M	fourth child
Geagan	Mrs. Michael	4271	26-Oct-1867	M	fifth pregnancy
Geary	Mrs.	150	08-Jun-1835		"This lady previous to her confinement was affected with giddiness & loss of sight at night."
Geary	Mrs. M.	504	25-Jun-1840	F	
Geede	Mrs. Richard	1422	16-Apr-1847	F	born a little after 5 AM
Gees	Mrs. Andrew	4286	08-Dec-1867	M	second pregnancy
Gees	Mrs. B. F.	2916	14-Jun-1857	F	third child
Gees	Mrs. B. F.	3617	20-Feb-1862	F	fifth child
Gees	Mrs. B. F.	3923	13-Sep-1864	F	first pregnancy
Gees	Mrs. B. F.	4110	23-Jun-1866	F	second pregnancy
Gees	Mrs. Franklin	2639	18-Aug-1855	M	second child
Gees	Mrs. G. F.	3217	23-Mar-1859	F	fourth child
Gees	Mrs. Richard	1733	28-Jul-1849	F	born 6 PM
Gees	Mrs. Richard	2399	26-Feb-1854	M	tenth child
Gees	Mrs. Richard	2754	27-May-1856	M	11th child
Gees	Mrs. Richard	3205	07-Mar-1859	M	12th child

75

Obstetrical Casebooks of Dr. F. E. Chatard – an alternative genealogical resource 1829-1883

Geete	Mrs. George	2052	08-Nov-1851	F	ninth child
Gegan	Mrs. J.	762	20-Sep-1842	M	eighth child
Gegan	Mrs. Joseph	88	24-Nov-1833		first child, seven months, "... suffered greatly from the beginning of her pregnancy." Child dead
Gegan	Mrs. Joseph	121	14-Oct-1834	F	see 24 Nov 1833 [#88], second child, 5.5 lbs.
Gegan	Mrs. Joseph	182	16-Mar-1836	F	see 14 Oct 1834 [#121], third child
Gegan	Mrs. Joseph	454	07-Jan-1840	F	sixth child
Gegan	Mrs. Joseph	608	17-Jul-1841	M	seventh child
Gegan	Mrs. Joseph	1145	05-May-1845	M	ninth child
Gegan	Mrs. Joseph	1437	23-May-1847	M	tenth child
Gegan	Mrs. Joseph	1958	04-Mar-1851	F	12th child
Gegan	Mrs. Joseph	2226	05-Jan-1853	M	13th child
Gegan	Mrs. Joseph	2381	16-Jan-1854	F	14th child
Gehre	Mrs. Robert	4956	29-Nov-1874	M	second pregnancy, attended by midwife, forceps
Geneste	Mrs. L.	4979	14-May-1875	F	fourth pregnancy
George	Mrs. T. J.	4268	23-Oct-1867	F	first pregnancy, attended by Dr. Fulton
Gerke	Mrs. Charles	4762	16-Jun-1872	F	fourth pregnancy
Germlig	Mrs. T.	3482	28-Jan-1861	M	first child
Gettier	Mrs. A. J.	3768	09-Apr-1863	M	third pregnancy
Gettier	Mrs. A. J.	4575	23-Jul-1870	M	fifth pregnancy
Gibbons	Mrs. Wm.	1084	05-Dec-1844	F	fifth child
Gibney	Mrs. G. S.	2854	17-Jan-1857	M	third child
Gibney	Mrs. George	3235	18-May-1859	F	fourth child
Gibney	Mrs. Henry	4959	02-Dec-1874	M	third pregnancy, called in consultation, child dead
Gibson	Mrs. C. C.	1977	18-May-1851	F	fourth child
Gibson	Mrs. Charles	996	29-May-1844	F	second child

76

Obstetrical Casebooks of Dr. F. E. Chatard – an alternative genealogical resource 1829-1883

Gibson	Mrs. Charles	2857	01-Feb-1857	M	fourth child
Gibson	Mrs. Charles A.	2299	30-Jun-1853	M	second child
Gibson	Mrs. Edmund	410	25-Aug-1839	F	seventh child
Gibson	Mrs. Edmund	638	24-Sep-1841	F	born 10:30 PM
Gibson	Mrs. Frederick	4218	08-May-1867	F	first pregnancy
Gibson	Mrs. Frederick	4745	17-Apr-1872	M	second pregnancy, forceps delivery, mother had convulsions
Gibson, Jr.	Mrs. G. S.	3467	19-Dec-1860	M	first child
Giese, Jr	Mrs. George	984	09-Apr-1844	F	third child
Gilder	Mrs. W. H.	2946	09-Aug-1857	M	first child
Gile	Mrs. George M.	668	06-Jan-1842	M	third child
Giles	Mrs. J. R.	646	25-Oct-1841	F	third child
Giles	Mrs. J. R.	902	13-Oct-1843	F	fourth child
Giles	Mrs. J. R.	1609	03-Aug-1848	F	born 5 AM
Giles	Mrs. J. R.	1895	28-Sep-1850	M	seventh child
Giles	Mrs. John R.	30-Jul-1846	F		fourth child
Giles	Mrs. John R.	305	20-Jun-1838	F	first child
Giles	Mrs. W. F.		20-Aug-1840	M	seventh child
Giles	Mrs. W. F.	322	09-Aug-1838		still born
Giles	Mrs. W. F.	398	20-Jul-1839	M	sixth child
Giles	Mrs. W. F.	852	22-May-1843	M	ninth child
Giles	Mrs. W. F.	951	22-Jan-1844	M	premature labor, child dead
Giles	Mrs. W. F.	1625	03-Oct-1848	M	first child
Giles	Mrs. W. F.	1844	23-May-1850	F	second child

Obstetrical Casebooks of Dr. F. E. Chatard – an alternative genealogical resource 1829-1883

	Given Name	Number	Date	Sex	Comments
Giles	Mrs. W. F.	2292	08-Jun-1853	M	third child
Giles	Mrs. W. F.	2665	04-Oct-1855	F	fourth child
Gill	Mrs. G. M.	1274	21-Apr-1846	F	born about 4 PM
Gill	Mrs. George	2394	12-Feb-1854	F	eighth child
Gill	Mrs. George M.	77	30-Jun-1833	F	second child
Gill	Mrs. George M.	462	14-Feb-1840	F	second child
Gill	Mrs. George M.	1715	09-Jun-1849	M	sixth child
Gill	Mrs. George M.	2045	24-Oct-1851	F	sixth child
Gill	Mrs. Wly	4316	16-Mar-1868	M	first pregnancy
Gill [McGill]	Mrs. Wm. G.	289	13-Mar-1838	F	first child
Gillan	Mrs. James	2750	20-May-1856	M	first child
Gillen	Mrs. James	3146	14-Oct-1858	F	third child
Gilman	Mrs.	108	15-Jun-1834		abortion at six weeks
Gilmor	Mrs. C.	541	08-Nov-1840	M	born 10 AM
Gilmor	Mrs. Charles	802	01-Jan-1843	M	second child
Gilmor	Mrs. Charles S.	2156	14-Jul-1852	M	third child
Gilmor	Mrs. J.	1427	30-Apr-1847	M	first child
Gilmor	Mrs. James D.	1700	08-Apr-1849	M	second child
Gilmor	Mrs. W.	1316	13-Aug-1846	M	third child
Gilmor	Mrs. William	1137	29-Mar-1845	M	second child
Gilmor	Mrs. William	1978	22-May-1851	F	fourth child
Gilmor	Mrs. William	2208	20-Nov-1852	M	fifth child
Gilmor	Mrs. Wm.	931	10-Dec-1843	M	first child

Obstetrical Casebooks of Dr. F. E. Chatard – an alternative genealogical resource 1829-1883

Gilmore	Mrs. Charles	1680	25-Feb-1849	F	first child
Gilmore	Mrs. James D.	2002	16-Jul-1851	F	third child
Gilmour	Mrs. Andrew	2797	02-Sep-1856	M	fifth child
Gilmour	Mrs. Charles	1893	26-Sep-1850	M	second child
Gilmour	Mrs. James D.	2223	21-Dec-1852	F	fourth child
Gilmour	Mrs. James D.	3047	21-Feb-1858	M	sixth child
Gilmour	Mrs. James D.	3291	10-Nov-1859	M	seventh child
Gilpin	Mrs. Matley	1825	25-Feb-1850	M	third child
Gist	Mrs.	1445	12-Jun-1847	M	second child
Gittings	Mrs. James	2970	25-Sep-1857	M	third child
Gittings	Mrs. James	3415	09-Sep-1860	F	fourth child
Gittings	Mrs. Richard	3067	06-Apr-1858	F	first child
Gittings	Mrs. Richard	3355	23-Mar-1860	M	second child
Gittings	Mrs. Richard	3529	07-Jun-1861	M	third child
Gittings	Mrs. Richard	3764	03-Apr-1863	F	fourth pregnancy
Gittings	Mrs. Richard	4002	11-May-1865	F	fifth pregnancy
Gittings	Mrs. Richard	4372	07-Sep-1868	F	sixth pregnancy
Gittings	Mrs. Richard	4604	01-Nov-1870	M	seventh pregnancy
Gittings	Mrs. Richard	4803	10-Dec-1872	F	eighth pregnancy
Gittings	Mrs. Richard	5180	11-Feb-1879	F	ninth pregnancy
Givens	Mrs. John C.	3346	04-Mar-1860	M	first child
Gleninger	Mrs. J. R.	3632	30-Apr-1862	M	born 10:45 PM
Gleninger	Mrs. John R.	3363	08-May-1860	M	first child
Godwin	Mrs.	1709	19-May-1849	M	third child
Golden	Mrs. J. C.	1197	25-Aug-1845	F	first child
Golden	Mrs. James C.	1446	20-Jun-1847	M	second child

79

Obstetrical Casebooks of Dr. F. E. Chatard – an alternative genealogical resource 1829-1883

Golden	Mrs. James C.	2701	13-Jan-1856	F	sixth child
Golder	Mrs. J. C.	1821	22-Feb-1850	M	third child
Golder	Mrs. Thomas	1952	26-Feb-1851	F	first child
Goldsborough	Mrs.	720	25-May-1842	M	fourth child
Goldsborough	Mrs.	1068	01-Nov-1844	M	fifth child, forceps delivery
Goldsborough	Mrs. Emily	1640	03-Nov-1848	F	colored, first child
Goldsborough	Mrs. N.	1518	28-Dec-1847	M	sixth child
Goldsborough	Mrs. R. H.	4648	31-Mar-1871	M	first pregnancy
Goldsbury	Emily	3119	26-Aug-1858		colored, consultation with Dr Frick and Dr Van Bibber, child dead
Gonder	Mrs.	1753	23-Sep-1849	F	First child
Gonley	Mrs. L.	1736	10-Aug-1849	F	born 3 AM
Gonley [Gonby]	Mrs. Louis	1378	17-Jan-1847	F	third child
Goode	Mrs.	1470	23-Aug-1847	M	first child
Goodwin	Mrs.	1889	13-Sep-1850	F	fourth child
Goodwin	Mrs.	2305	14-Jul-1853	F	fifth child
Goodwin	Mrs. Thomas	2620	15-Jul-1855	F	seventh child
Goodwin	Mrs. Thomas	3045	21-Feb-1858	F	seventh child
Gordon	Mrs. Alexander	569	25-Jan-1841	F	first child
Gordon	Mrs. Alexander	963	17-Feb-1844	M	third child, mother died on 22 February
Gordon	Mrs. Basil	1064	26-Oct-1844	M	third child
Gordon	Mrs. Douglass	4148	05-Oct-1866	M	sixth pregnancy
Gordon	Mrs. Douglass	4417	07-Feb-1869	F	seventh pregnancy
Gordon	Mrs. John M.	756	03-Sep-1842	F	fifth child
Gorman	Mrs. P.	4763	29-Jun-1872	F	third pregnancy
Gorman	Mrs. Patrick	4393	10-Dec-1868	M	first pregnancy

Obstetrical Casebooks of Dr. F. E. Chatard – an alternative genealogical resource 1829-1883

Gorsuch	Mrs. J. J.	3270	11-Sep-1859	F	first child
Gorsuch	Mrs. J. T.	3586	11-Nov-1861	F	second child
Gorsuch	Mrs. J. T.	4645	03-Mar-1871	M	seventh pregnancy
Gorsuch	Mrs. J. T.	4914	08-Jul-1874	M	"This lady's previous labours have generally been very tedious & difficult … this time the labor was rapid
Gorsuch	Mrs. J. W.	4558	11-Jun-1870	F	first pregnancy
Gorsuch	Mrs. James	4518	27-Dec-1869	M	first pregnancy
Gorsuch	Mrs. John T.	3863	07-Mar-1864	M	third pregnancy
Gorsuch	Mrs. John T.	4128	03-Aug-1866	M	fourth pregnancy. "She was very ill after her confinement and her recovery was very slow."
Gorsuch	Mrs. John T.	4267	22-Oct-1867	F	fifth pregnancy
Gorsuch	Mrs. John T.	4388	21-Nov-1868	F	sixth pregnancy
Gorsuch	Mrs. John T.	4828	08-Apr-1873	M	eighth pregnancy
Gorsuch	Mrs. P.	601	07-Jun-1841	F	born 1:30 AM
Gorsuch	Mrs. P.	861	24-Jun-1843	M	born 6 AM
Gorsuch	Mrs. P.	1125	14-Feb-1845	M	ninth child
Gorsuch	Mrs. P.	1345	15-Oct-1846	M	tenth child
Gorsuch	Mrs. Peregrin	2027	09-Sep-1851	F	11th child
Gorsuch	Mrs. Peregrine	1681	25-Feb-1849	M	11th child
Gorsuch	Mrs. Peregrine	2529	19-Dec-1854	M	13th child
Gorsuch	Mrs. S. W.	4770	17-Jul-1872		second child
Gosnall	Mrs. Richard	2612	02-Jul-1855	M	fourth child
Gosnall	Mrs. Richard	3012	02-Dec-1857	F	fourth child
Gosnall	Mrs. Richard	3342	23-Feb-1860	F	fifth child
Gosnall	Mrs. Richard	3634	04-May-1862	F	sixth child

Obstetrical Casebooks of Dr. F. E. Chatard – an alternative genealogical resource 1829-1883

Gosnell	Mrs.	1338	23-Sep-1846	M	first child
Gosnell [?]	Mrs. Richard	2281	12-May-1853	F	second child
Gossage	Mrs.	2357	18-Nov-1853	F	seventh child, seven months, child dead
Gossery	Mrs. Hugh	5079	15-Sep-1876	F	first pregnancy
Gottlieb	Mrs. F. H.	5134	01-Jul-1877	F	first pregnancy
Govans	Mrs.	10		F	first child, the child died on the fifth or sixth day
Govans	Mrs.	69	12-Mar-1833	M	see Jan 1830 [#10]; second child. "It was a very large child." Child died six days later. Long description of care.
Gowland	Mrs.	1528	14-Jan-1848	M	fifth child
Grady	Mrs.	471	21-Mar-1840	F	fifth child
Grady	Mrs. James	729	27-Jun-1842	F	sixth child
Grady	Mrs. James	1536	29-Jan-1848	M	born 10:30 AM
Grafflin	Mrs. Joseph	4364	15-Aug-1868	M	sixth pregnancy
Grant	Mrs.	483	24-Apr-1840	F	fifth child
Grant	Mrs. Edward	3003	15-Nov-1857	F	second child
Grant	Mrs. Edward	3236	20-May-1859	F	third child
Grant	Mrs. Edward	3496	25-Feb-1861	F	fifth child
Grant	Mrs. Edward	3639	20-May-1862	M	fifth child
Grant	Mrs. Edward B.	2714	15-Feb-1856	F	first child
Graves	Mrs.	245	21-Aug-1837	F	fifth child
Graves	Ruth	1940	30-Jan-1851	F/F	colored, attended by Dr Coulburn, twins
Gray	Mrs.	2459	07-Aug-1854	F	third child
Gray	Mrs. Barney	2496	09-Oct-1854	F	fifth child
Gray	Mrs. Bernard	1916	19-Nov-1850	M	third child. It died a few hours after.
Gray	Mrs. Bernard	2087	22-Jan-1852	M	fourth child

Obstetrical Casebooks of Dr. F. E. Chatard – an alternative genealogical resource 1829-1883

Gray	Mrs. Bernard	2878	12-Mar-1857	F	eighth child
Gray	Mrs. Bernard	3386	22-Jun-1860	M	eighth child, child dead
Gray	Mrs. Bernard	3666	08-Aug-1862	F	ninth child
Gray	Mrs. David	3562	26-Aug-1861	M	third child
Gray	Mrs. David	4004	12-May-1865	F	fourth pregnancy
Gray	Mrs. David W.	3062	29-Mar-1858	M	second child
Gray	Mrs. Hugh	3536	23-Jun-1861	F	fifth child
Gray	Mrs. J. T.	3864	07-Mar-1864	F	ninth pregnancy
Green	Mrs.	181	17-Feb-1836		born at 6 AM
Green	Mrs.	3730	04-Jan-1863	M	at St. Vincent's Asylum, first child
Green	Mrs. C. Bennett	2943	28-Jul-1857	F	fifth child
Green	Mrs. Samuel	3125	02-Sep-1858	M	third child
Green	Mrs. Sarah	298	23-Apr-1838	M	third child, previous were stillborn
Greenwell	Mrs. J. C.	3572	27-Sep-1861	M	second child
Greenwell	Mrs. J. C◇	3398	23-Jul-1860	M	first child
Greve	Mrs. J. J.	2986	24-Oct-1857	M	third child
Grey	Mrs. Bernard	1620	24-Sep-1848	F	first child
Grey	Mrs. Bernard	3818	09-Nov-1863	M	tenth pregnancy
Grey	Mrs. Bernard	4048	06-Nov-1865	M	11th pregnancy
Griffis	Mrs. Thomas J.	4220	18-May-1867	F	seventh pregnancy
Griffin	Mrs. Edward	3621	17-Mar-1862	F	first child
Griffith	Mrs.	139	19-Mar-1835	F	first child
Griffith	Mrs. C.	226	07-Mar-1837	F	second child, mother died 11 March at 12 o'clock PM
Grimes	Mrs. J. A.	2825	15-Nov-1855	M	seventh child
Grinnell	Mrs. C. A.	773	03-Nov-1842	F	second child

83

Obstetrical Casebooks of Dr. F. E. Chatard – an alternative genealogical resource 1829-1883

Grinold	Mrs.	297	19-Apr-1838	F	14th child
Griswold	Mrs. B. B.	2203	10-Nov-1852	M	second child
Griswold	Mrs. B. B.	2462	16-Aug-1854		third child. "The child was born during my engagement with the above call."
Griswold	Mrs. D.	413	04-Sep-1839	M	15th child, 10 pounds
Groeninger	Mrs. John	2306	14-Jul-1853	F	first child
Groeninger	Mrs. John	2734	07-Apr-1856	F	second child
Groner	Mrs.	4357	03-Aug-1868	M	first pregnancy
Grove	Mrs. Caroline	2482	19-Sep-1854	M	first child
Grove	Mrs. J. J.	2713	13-Feb-1856	M	second child
Grove	Mrs. J. J.	3300	07-Dec-1859	F	fourth child
Guerand	Mrs.	1397	16-Feb-1847	F	forceps delivery
Guest	Mrs.	1056	17-Oct-1844	M	second child, died after a few hours
Guest	Mrs. G.	4241	11-Aug-1867	M	third pregnancy
Guilfoy	Mrs. T.	4519	01-Jan-1870	M	first pregnancy
Guillin	Mrs. Victor	3796	30-Jul-1863	M	first pregnancy
Gump	Mrs. Jacob	4902	14-May-1874	F	first pregnancy
Gwynn	Mrs.	118	10-Sep-1834	F	ninth child
Gwynn	Mrs. R.	1457	31-Jul-1847	M	first child
Hains	Mrs. Peter	4732	09-Jan-1872	M	third pregnancy
Hall	Mrs. Blanche	2408	26-Mar-1854	M	first child
Hall	Mrs. C. G.	3268	05-Sep-1859	M	first child, attended by Dr. Patterson
Hall	Mrs. Levi	3798	01-Aug-1863	M	fourth pregnancy
Hall	Mrs. Thomas	1471	24-Aug-1847	M	eighth child
Hammond	Mrs. A.	5148	10-Sep-1877	M	second pregnancy, forceps delivery
Hammond	Mrs. Charles	3524	17-May-1861	F	third child

Obstetrical Casebooks of Dr. F. E. Chatard – an alternative genealogical resource 1829-1883

Hammond	Mrs. Charles	3713	13-Dec-1862	F	fourth child
Hammond	Mrs. Charles	4150	08-Oct-1866		fifth pregnancy, seven months. "This patient had been suffering for some days with pain in the head and swelling of the face & extremities." child dead
Hammond	Mrs. Charles	4880	23-Jan-1874	M	seventh pregnancy
Hammond	Mrs. Charles H.	3098	26-Jun-1858	M	first child
Hammond	Mrs. Charles H.	3282	19-Oct-1859	M	second child
Hammond	Mrs. Charles H.	4337	28-May-1868	M	sixth pregnancy
Hammond	Mrs. W. A.	5240	09-Aug-1881	F	fourth pregnancy
Hammond	Mrs. Wm. A.	4798	25-Nov-1872	M	first pregnancy
Hammond	Mrs. Wm. A.	5191	27-May-1879	M	third pregnancy, "She was very feeble & had great nausea & vomiting, which I attributed to the effect of the chloroform administered during the last stages of labor."
Hampson	Mrs. A. J.	4633	15-Jan-1871	M	first pregnancy, aged 40 years. "She had a long & tedious labor." Child lived only a few hours. Complicated course, she died on the 31st
Hampson	Mrs. J.	3999	04-May-1865	F	second pregnancy
Hanan	Mrs. John	4352	17-Jul-1868	F	third pregnancy
Hananay	Mrs. Patrick	2341	05-Oct-1853	F	first child
Hanaway	Mrs. Bridget	2605	11-Jun-1855	M	second child
Hanaway	Mrs. Bridget	3163	18-Nov-1858	F	third child
Hanaway	Mrs. Patrick	3703	11-Nov-1862	F	fourth child
Handrahar	Mrs. Brien	2784	19-Aug-1856	M	first child
Handy	Mrs.	1300	29-Jun-1846	F	second child
Haney	Mrs.	1540	04-Feb-1848	M	born 3 AM
Haney	Mrs. Daniel	5228	29-Nov-1880	F	first pregnancy aged 35, forceps delivery
Haney	Mrs. J. G.	2562	27-Feb-1855	F	second child

Obstetrical Casebooks of Dr. F. E. Chatard – an alternative genealogical resource 1829-1883

Hanlan	Mrs. Sarah	1824	25-Feb-1850	M	first child
Hanley	Mrs. Patrick	3365	13-May-1860	M	first child
Hannah	Mrs.	1037	10-Sep-1844	F	fifth child
Hanse	Mrs. O.P.	683	14-Feb-1842	M	first child, stillborn
Hanzsche	Mrs. Edward	2968	22-Sep-1857	M	first child
Hanzsche	Mrs. Edward	3368	18-May-1860	M	second child
Hanzsche	Mrs. Edward	3928	22-Sep-1864	M	third pregnancy
Hanzsche	Mrs. Edward	4211	24-Apr-1867	F	fourth pregnancy
Hanzsche	Mrs. F.	3197	19-Feb-1859	F	third child
Hanzsche	Mrs. F.	3470	26-Dec-1860	F	fourth child, "… it lived only a few hours."
Hanzsche	Mrs. Frederick	2497	11-Oct-1854	M	first child
Hanzsche	Mrs. Frederick	2869	01-Mar-1857	M	third child
Hanzsche	Mrs. Frederick	3588	13-Nov-1861	F	fifth child. "The child died a few hours after her birth & very unexpectedly."
Hardenbrock	Mrs. J.	4258	22-Sep-1867	M	third pregnancy
Hardenbrock	Mrs. J. A.	4031	15-Sep-1865	M	second pregnancy
Hardesty	Mrs.	513	27-Jul-1840	F	fifth child
Hardesty	Mrs.	4042	24-Oct-1865	F	child born at 4;20 AM
Hardesty	Mrs. R. C.	4230	29-Jun-1867	F	third pregnancy
Hardesty	Mrs. R. S.	549	27-Nov-1840	M	third child
Hardesty	Mrs. R. S.	806	08-Jan-1843	M	fourth child
Hardesty	Mrs. Richard	1527	13-Jan-1848	F	seventh child
Hardesty	Mrs. Richard S.	1074	15-Nov-1844	M	fifth child
Hardisty	Mrs. Henry	2245	21-Feb-1853	M	seventh child
Harig	Mrs. Bernard	2945	03-Aug-1857	M	ninth child
Harman	Mrs. Joseph	1491	14-Oct-1847	F	first child

Obstetrical Casebooks of Dr. F. E. Chatard – an alternative genealogical resource 1829-1883

Harman	Mrs. Samuel	76	30-Jun-1833	F	first child
Harmon	Mrs. George	23	14-Jun-1831	M	first child, "Tall & well formed, has enjoyed very good health." eight pounds
Harrigan	Mrs. Thomas	4158	18-Nov-1866	M	first pregnancy. "The child was feeble and died about two weeks after birth."
Harrington	Mrs. Abraham	3614	09-Feb-1862	F	third child
Harrington	Mrs. Abraham	3835	03-Jan-1864	M	fourth pregnancy
Harrington	Mrs. Abraham	4069	04-Jan-1866	M	fourth pregnancy
Harrington	Mrs. S.	2271	25-Apr-1853	M	ninth child
Harris	Mrs. Alexander	3231	11-May-1859	M	fifth child
Harris	Mrs. D. C.	794	17-Dec-1842	M	first child
Harris	Mrs. Thomas	3449	27-Nov-1860	M	fifth child
Harris	Mrs. W. C.	137	19-Feb-1835	M	born 4:30 PM
Harris	Mrs. W. C.	229	27-Mar-1837	F	born at one o'clock PM
Harris	Mrs. W. Hall	5197	03-Aug-1879	M	second pregnancy
Harris	Mrs. W. Hall	5233	01-Mar-1881	M	third pregnancy
Harris	Mrs. W. Hall	5155	06-Apr-1878	F	first pregnancy
Harrison	Mrs. C.	4624	15-Dec-1870	F	second pregnancy
Harrison	Mrs. Charles	4259	25-Sep-1867	M	first pregnancy
Harrison	Mrs. Frederick	640	08-Oct-1841	F	second child
Harrison	Mrs. Frederick	952	23-Jan-1844	M	third child
Harrison	Mrs. Frederick	1384	27-Jan-1847	M	fourth child
Harrison	Mrs. Frederick	2090	25-Jan-1852	F	sixth child
Harrison	Mrs. G. L.	1546	26-Feb-1848	F	second child
Harrison	Mrs. George	1346	20-Oct-1846	F	first child
Harrison	Mrs. George	3203	02-Mar-1859	F	third child

Obstetrical Casebooks of Dr. F. E. Chatard – an alternative genealogical resource 1829-1883

Harrison	Mrs. George L.	1820	22-Feb-1850	F	third child
Harrison	Mrs. George L.	2988	25-Oct-1857	F	second child
Harrison	Mrs. George L.	3483	31-Jan-1861	M	fourth child
Harrison	Mrs. George L.	4047	05-Nov-1865	F	fifth pregnancy
Harrison	Mrs. George L.	4710	28-Nov-1871	M	sixth pregnancy
Harrison	Mrs. John B.	5232	24-Jan-1881	M	first pregnancy, forceps delivery
Harrison	Mrs. John B.	5244	19-Jan-1882	M	second pregnancy
Harrison	Mrs. M.	4426	07-Mar-1869	M	first pregnancy. "It was very feeble and died a few days after its birth."
Harrison	Mrs. Malory	4578	27-Jul-1870	M	second pregnancy, child was dead
Harrison	Mrs. W.	1072	12-Nov-1844	F	fifth child
Harrison	Mrs. W.	1495	21-Oct-1847	M	sixth child
Hart	Mrs. Archibald	1430	10-May-1847	M	second child
Hart	Mrs. Rich	3229	06-May-1859	M	seventh child
Hart	Mrs. Robert	1616	19-Sep-1848	F	third child
Hartings	Mrs. Joseph S.	1398	17-Feb-1847	M	second child
Hartmyer	Mrs. Henry	4318	23-Mar-1868	M	first pregnancy
Hartzell	Mrs.	525	25-Sep-1840	M	twin boys, 7 months
Harvey	Mrs. Charles	1356	25-Nov-1846	F	second child
Harvey	Mrs. Charles	1587	20-Jun-1848	M	third child
Harvey	Mrs. Charles	1778	27-Nov-1849	M	fourth child
Harvey	Mrs. Charles	1991	18-Jun-1851	F	fifth child
Harvey	Mrs. Charles	2212	28-Nov-1852	M	sixth child
Harvey	Mrs. Charles	2441	24-Jun-1854	M	second child
Harvey	Mrs. Charles	2763	21-Jun-1856	M	tenth child
Harvey	Mrs. Charles	2972	05-Oct-1857	M	11th child, Dr Dunbar attended
Harvey	Mrs. Charles	3393	11-Jul-1860	M	tenth child

Obstetrical Casebooks of Dr. F. E. Chatard – an alternative genealogical resource 1829-1883

Harvey	Mrs. Harry D.	1284	25-May-1846	M	sixth child
Harvey	Mrs. Henry	1742	08-Sep-1849	M	eighth child
Harvey	Mrs. Henry	2126	21-Apr-1852	F	ninth child
Harvey	Mrs. Henry D.	1530	17-Jan-1848	F	seventh child
Harwood	Mrs.	507	05-Jul-1840	M	fifth child, 9.5 pounds
Haskins	Mrs. Moses	2928	02-Jul-1857	F	colored, first child
Haskins	Mrs. Thomas	1465	13-Aug-1847	F	first child, stillborn, forceps delivery
Hasson	Mrs. P.	320	02-Aug-1838	M	second child
Hasting	Mrs. J. S.	1718	29-Jun-1849	F	third child
Hastings	Mrs. J. S.	2150	18-Jun-1852	F	premature birth 4 months
Hastings	Mrs. Joseph S.	2295	12-Jun-1853	M	born 1:30 PM
Hastings	Mrs. Joseph S.	2711	09-Feb-1856	F	born 1:30 PM
Hastings	Mrs. Joseph S.	2917	15-Jun-1857	F	born about 2:10 AM
Hastings	Mrs. Joseph S.	3212	09-Mar-1859	F	seventh child
Hastings	Mrs. Joseph S.	3571	21-Sep-1861	M	eighth child
Hastings	Mrs. Joseph S.	3724	29-Dec-1862	M	ninth child
Hastings, Jr.	Mrs. Joseph	1172	04-Jul-1845	M	first child
Haswell	Mrs.	1209	01-Oct-1845	M	first child
Haupt	Mrs.	120	12-Oct-1834	M	second child
Haupt	Mrs.	216	15-Nov-1836	M	third child
Hawley	Mrs. R. K.	1989	18-Jun-1851	F	second child
Hayden	Mrs. J. F.	3204	06-Mar-1859	F	second child
Hayden	Mrs. J. F.	4897	17-Apr-1874	M	fifth pregnancy, stillborn
Hayden	Mrs. John	4304	08-Feb-1868	F	second pregnancy
Haydon	Mrs. J. F.	2901	12-May-1857	M	first child
Haye	Mrs. Edward	3490	15-Feb-1861	M	second child

Obstetrical Casebooks of Dr. F. E. Chatard – an alternative genealogical resource 1829-1883

Hayes	Mrs. J. S.	5017	15-Nov-1875	F	sixth pregnancy
Hayes	Mrs. J. S.	5167	26-Aug-1878	F	eighth pregnancy
Hayes	Mrs. John	5145	28-Aug-1877	M	seventh pregnancy
Hayes	Mrs. John S.	5227	17-Nov-1880	M	ninth pregnancy
Hayne	Mrs. Charles	2413	19-Apr-1854	M	fifth child
Hayne	Mrs. Charles	2803	07-Oct-1856	M	sixth child
Haynes	Mrs. Charles	2044	22-Oct-1851	F	fourth child
Haynes	Mrs. Charles	3182	13-Jan-1859	M	born 2:30 AM
Haynes	Mrs. Charles	3548	04-Aug-1861	M	tenth child
Haynes	Mrs. Charles	3794	21-Jul-1863	M	tenth pregnancy
Hays	Mrs.	503	22-Jun-1840	F	first child
Hays	Mrs.	820	14-Feb-1843	M	first child
Hazel	Mrs.	146	16-May-1835	F	sixth child
Hazelhurst	Mrs. Henry	2467	24-Aug-1854	F	first child
Hazelhurst	Mrs. Henry	2684	28-Nov-1855	M	second child
Hazelhurst	Mrs. Henry	3011	01-Dec-1857	F	third child
Heald	Mrs. Howard	3081	06-May-1858	F	second child
Heald	Mrs. Howard	3510	21-Apr-1861	M	third child
Heald	Mrs. J. R.	2396	21-Feb-1854	M	second child
Heald	Mrs. W. H.	1134	02-Mar-1845	F	first child
Healy	Mrs. John	2641	21-Aug-1855	M	first child
Healy	Mrs. John	3667	11-Aug-1862	M	first child
Heath	Mrs.	451	06-Jan-1840	F	
Hechenthall	Mrs. Louis M.	2771	20-Jul-1856	F	first child
Heffern	Mrs. Hugh	3502	23-Mar-1861	F	first child

Obstetrical Casebooks of Dr. F. E. Chatard – an alternative genealogical resource 1829-1883

Heighe	Mrs. B. C.	1669	05-Feb-1849	M	ninth child
Heighe	Mrs. B. M.	2088	22-Jan-1852	M	ninth child
Heiskell	Mrs. Muroe [?]	4512	15-Dec-1869	M	second pregnancy
Hellen	Mrs. H.	2161	27-Jul-1852	F	fourth child
Heller	Mrs. H.	1716	21-Jun-1849	F	second child
Hellone [?]	Mrs. James	3069	07-Apr-1858	F	second child
Hemmick	Mrs. Wm.	2344	09-Oct-1853	M	born 3 AM
Henderson	Mrs.	526	29-Sep-1840	F	third child
Henderson	Mrs. Henry	738	20-Jul-1842	F	fourth child
Henderson	Mrs. J. A.	4746	17-Apr-1872	M	first pregnancy, "The child had quite a large head."
Henlon	Mrs. Bernard	3932	03-Oct-1864	F	third pregnancy
Henry	Mrs.	2351	08-Nov-1853	M/	second child, twins
Henry	Mrs. Dr. S. H.	1192	16-Aug-1845	M	first child
Hering	Mrs. Alfred	3800	10-Aug-1863	F	first pregnancy
Herman	Mrs. C. C.	3641	22-May-1862	F	fourth child
Herman	Mrs. C. C.	5188	30-Apr-1879	F	first pregnancy, forceps delivery
Herman	Mrs. Christopher	2632	12-Aug-1855	F	second child
Herman	Mrs. Christopher	3367	18-May-1860	F	third child
Herman	Mrs. H. W.	4423	01-Mar-1869	M	first pregnancy
Herman	Mrs. H. W.	4569	06-Jul-1870	M	second pregnancy
Herman	Mrs. H. W.	4953	19-Nov-1874	F	fifth pregnancy
Herman	Mrs. H. W.	5075	12-Aug-1875	F	sixth pregnancy
Herman	Mrs. W. H.	4708	26-Nov-1871	F	third pregnancy
Hern	Mrs.	3527	26-May-1861	M	seventh child

Obstetrical Casebooks of Dr. F. E. Chatard – an alternative genealogical resource 1829-1883

Herr	Mrs. John	875	10-Aug-1843	F	first child
Herr	Mrs. John	1041	15-Sep-1844	M	second child
Herr	Mrs. John	1307	16-Jul-1846	M	third child
Herzog	Mrs. John	2404	19-Mar-1854	F	second child
Herzog	Mrs. John	4862	23-Oct-1873	M	eighth pregnancy
Herzog	Mrs. John	5171	22-Oct-1878	F	ninth pregnancy
Heslip	Mrs.	1648	25-Nov-1848	M	first child
Hess	Mrs. Frank W.	4549	15-May-1870	M	fourth pregnancy, forceps delivery, "The child was born at 410 am it was feeble & had all the appearance of a 7 month child and died."
Heuisler	Mrs. Stanislaus	2378	11-Jan-1854	M	first child
Heuisler	Mrs. Stanislaus	2740	23-Apr-1856	F	second child
Heuisler	Mrs. Stanislaus	3097	25-Jun-1858	M	third child
Heuisler	Mrs. Stanislaus	3432	23-Oct-1860	M	fourth child
Heuser	Mrs. Dr. Charles	2898	10-May-1857	F	first child
Hewlett	Mrs. James	2960	11-Sep-1857	M	first child
Hezlip	Mrs. N.	1925	06-Dec-1850	M	second child
Hiblith	Mrs. Patrick	3958	13-Dec-1864	F	sixth pregnancy
Hickey	Mrs. C. F.	5080	21-Sep-1876	M	first pregnancy, "The child was born before I arrived. It was stillborn."
Hickey	Mrs. Ed.	4513	16-Dec-1869	F	second pregnancy
Hickey	Mrs. Edward	4219	11-May-1867	F	first pregnancy
Hickey	Mrs. Edward	4751	28-Apr-1872	F	third pregnancy
Hickey	Mrs. Edward	4971	04-Feb-1875	M	fourth pregnancy
Hickey	Mrs. Edward B.	5086	21-Oct-1876	F	fifth pregnancy
Hickey	Mrs. James	954	28-Jan-1844	M	second child, "the child was large & strong"
Hickey	Mrs. James	1662	13-Jan-1849	M	fifth child

Obstetrical Casebooks of Dr. F. E. Chatard – an alternative genealogical resource 1829-1883

Hickey	Mrs. James	1816	15-Feb-1850	M	sixth child
Hickey	Mrs. Jonas	717	15-May-1842	M	first child
Hickley	Mrs.	396	13-Jul-1839	F	first child
Hickley	Mrs.	573	01-Feb-1841	M	second child
Hickley	Mrs. R. J.	823	23-Feb-1843	M	third child
Hickley	Mrs. R. J.	1013	12-Jul-1844	M	fourth child
Hickley	Mrs. R. J.	1352	04-Nov-1846	M	fifth child
Hicky	Mrs. James	1343	13-Oct-1846	M	fourth child
Higgenbothom	Mrs. John	1028	25-Aug-1844	M	first child
Higginbothim	Mrs. John	3566	07-Sep-1861	F	eighth child
Higginbothom	Mrs. John	3134	27-Sep-1858	M	seventh child
Higginbothom	Mrs. John	1295	21-Jun-1846	M	second child
Higginbothom	Mrs. John	1539	02-Feb-1848	M	third child
Higginbothom	Mrs. John	1785	11-Dec-1849	F	fourth child
Higginbothom	Mrs. John	2098	08-Feb-1852	M	fifth child
Higginbothom	Mrs. John	2707	05-Feb-1856	M	sixth child
Higginbothom	Mrs. John	3881	19-Apr-1864	M	ninth pregnancy
Higgins	Mrs.	157	18-Aug-1835	M	third child
Hilker	Mrs. Henry G.	5094	20-Dec-1876	F	first pregnancy
Hilker	Mrs. Solomon	2388	29-Jan-1854	F	third child
Hill	Mrs. W. B.	2229	14-Jan-1853	M	first child
Hillartin	Mrs. J. H.	3952	06-Dec-1864	M	first pregnancy
Hillen	Mrs. Solomon	2585	15-Apr-1855	F	fourth child
Hillen	Mrs. Solomon	3170	07-Dec-1858	M	fifth child
Hillen, Jr.	Mrs.	1708	19-May-1849	M	attended by Dr. Yates
Hillen, Jr.	Mrs. S. A.	1386	28-Jan-1847	F	first child

93

Obstetrical Casebooks of Dr. F. E. Chatard – an alternative genealogical resource 1829-1883

Hillinghirst	Mrs. A.	4254	12-Sep-1867	M	first pregnancy
Hilzer	Mrs. A.	4382	08-Nov-1868	M	first pregnancy
Hinard	Mrs. Joshua	1668	05-Feb-1849	M	second child
Hincks	Mrs. C. D.	2675	29-Oct-1855	F	first child
Hinder	Mrs. Frederick	2141	31-May-1852	F	second child
Hines	Mrs.	706	13-Apr-1842	M	fifth child
Hines	Mrs. Patrick	4434	26-Mar-1869	F	ninth pregnancy
Hinrichs	Mrs. C.	4647	13-Mar-1871	F	sixth pregnancy
Hinrichs	Mrs. Charles	2589	27-Apr-1855	F	first child
Hinrichs	Mrs. Christophe	3327	18-Jan-1860	F	third child
Hinrichs	Mrs. Christophe	3990	10-Apr-1865	F	fifth pregnancy
Hinrichs	Mrs. Christopher	2766	09-Jul-1856	M	second child
Hinrichs	Mrs. Christopher	3762	26-Mar-1863	M	fourth pregnancy
Hinter	Mrs. Frederick	1630	13-Oct-1848	M	first child
Hiser	Mrs. H.	282	16-Feb-1838	F	second child, first born 22 Jan '36. Mother died
Hisler	Mrs.	12	12-Mar-1830	M	first child, nine pounds
Hisler	Mrs.	43	26-Jan-1832	M	see 12 Mar 1830. Second child, 9.5 pounds
Hisler	Mrs.	44	17-Feb-1832	M	mother-in-law of above [#43], tenth child
Hiss	Mrs. George	4843	30-Jun-1873	M	second pregnancy
Hiss	Mrs. George	4973	14-Mar-1875	M	third pregnancy
Hitchcock	Mrs. Wm.	3716	17-Dec-1862	F	second child
Hitzelberger	Mrs.	1650	29-Nov-1848	M	second child, stillborn
Hitzelberger	Mrs. Wm. G.	1703	23-Apr-1849	F	fifth child
Hobbitts	Mrs. Patrick	3615	10-Feb-1862	M	fifth child

94

Obstetrical Casebooks of Dr. F. E. Chatard – an alternative genealogical resource 1829-1883

Surname	First	Number	Date	Sex	Notes
Hoblits	Mrs. P.	4248	30-Aug-1867	F	seventh pregnancy
Hobson	Mrs. George W.	3604	07-Jan-1862	F	first child
Hodges	Mrs.	1541	05-Feb-1848	F	first child
Hodges	Mrs. George W.	4978	11-May-1875	M	second pregnancy, forceps delivery
Hodges	Mrs. Howard	4910	21-Jun-1874	M	first pregnancy, forceps delivery
Hodges	Mrs. T. Harris	1030	30-Aug-1844	F	second child
Hoffman	Mrs. G. B.	1021	10-Aug-1844	M	second child
Hoffman	Mrs. George P.	3058	17-Mar-1858	M	first child
Hoffman	Mrs. J. Latimer	2109	07-Mar-1852	M	second child
Hoffman	Mrs. Josiah	178	28-Jan-1836	M	first child, premature about eight months
Hoffman	Mrs. Roger	796	18-Dec-1842	M	third child
Hoffmann	Mrs. G. B.	713	06-May-1842	M	first child
Hoffmann	Mrs. Latimer	1751	22-Sep-1849	F	first child
Hoffmann	Mrs. Wm. Gilmour	2973	08-Oct-1857	F	first child
Hogg	Mrs. James	335	14-Sep-1838	F	first child, still born. Assisted Dr. P. Chatard
Holland	Mrs.	643	15-Oct-1841	F	second child
Holland	Mrs. John	2200	06-Nov-1852	M	second child
Hollen	Mrs. H.	1849	07-Jun-1850	F	third child
Holliday	Mrs. Lamar	4543	08-May-1870	F	second pregnancy
Hollins	George	488	09-May-1840	M	fourth child
Hollins	Mrs. Cumberland	1891	20-Sep-1850	F	first child
Hollins	Mrs. G.	306	22-Jun-1838	M	third child
Hollins	Mrs. G. N.	899	02-Oct-1843	M	sixth child
Hollins	Mrs. George	165	18-Nov-1835	M	second child

Obstetrical Casebooks of Dr. F. E. Chatard – an alternative genealogical resource 1829-1883

Holloaway	Mrs. J.	4131	09-Aug-1866	F	first pregnancy
Hollyday	Mrs.	1265	14-Mar-1846	M	the child being born when I arrived
Holmes	Mrs. John	4752	05-May-1872	M	third pregnancy, "Each of her previous labours were very severe, the 1st child was delivered with forceps & died a few days after, the 2nd presented the feet & died in the
Holmes	Mrs. William	4439	16-Apr-1869	F	second pregnancy
Holmes	Mrs. William	4609	14-Nov-1870	M	third pregnancy
Holmes	Mrs. William	4774	28-Aug-1872	F	fourth pregnancy
Holmes	Mrs. William	5216	13-Mar-1880	F	seventh pregnancy
Holmes	Mrs. Wm.	2195	24-Oct-1852	F	second child
Holmes	Mrs. Wm.	4247	29-Aug-1867	M	first pregnancy
Holmes	Mrs. Wm.	4927	28-Aug-1874	M	fifth pregnancy
Holmes	Mrs. Wm.	5152	18-Mar-1878	M	sixth pregnancy
Holtz	Mrs. E.	564	07-Jan-1841	M	fourth child
Homans	Mrs. J. Smith	1450	02-Jul-1847	F	The child was born soon after I entered the room
Honeywell	Mrs. C.	1488	07-Oct-1847	M	first child, stillborn
Honeywell	Mrs. C. B.	1743	09-Sep-1849	M	second child
Honeywell	Mrs. Charles	2165	05-Aug-1852	F	third child
Honeywell	Mrs. Charles	2554	03-Feb-1855	F	fourth child
Honeywell	Mrs. Charles	2935	11-Jul-1857	M	fifth child
Honeywell	Mrs. Charles	3329	24-Jan-1860	M	sixth child
Hooff	Mrs. I. I.	4456	22-May-1869	M	first pregnancy
Hooff	Mrs. J.	4592	30-Sep-1870	M	second pregnancy, seventh month
Hook	Mrs. Frederick	2075	18-Dec-1851	M	fourth child
Hook	Mrs. Frederick	2353	13-Nov-1853	F	fifth child
Hook	Mrs. Frederick	1344	13-Oct-1846	F	second child

96

Obstetrical Casebooks of Dr. F. F. Chatard – an alternative genealogical resource 1829-1883

Hooper	Mrs. I.	3943	10-Nov-1864	M	seventh pr
Hopkins	Mrs.	384	13-May-1839	M	first child
Hopkins	Mrs. J. Seth	4627	24-Dec-1870	F	first pregnancy
Hopkins	Mrs. J. Seth	5186	15-Apr-1879	F	third pregnancy
Hopkins	Mrs. James	2063	28-Nov-1851	F	first child
Hopkins	Mrs. James	2445	11-Jul-1854	F	third child
Hopkins	Mrs. Joseph	1642	12-Nov-1848	F	premature, 5-6 months
Hopkins	Mrs. Joseph	1801	26-Jan-1850	M	second child
Hopkins	Mrs. Joseph	2051	08-Nov-1851	F	second child
Hopkins	Mrs. Joseph	2366	15-Dec-1853	F/F	third child
Hopkins	Mrs. Joseph	2841	13-Dec-1856	M	fifth child
Hopkins	Mrs. Joseph	3186	20-Jan-1859	M	sixth child
Hopkins	Mrs. Joseph	3434	27-Oct-1860	F	seventh child
Hopkins	Mrs. Joseph	3702	08-Nov-1862	M	eighth child
Hopkins	Mrs. L. N.	1281	14-May-1846	F	fifth child
Hopkins	Mrs. Lambert	855	13-Jun-1843	F	fourth child
Hopkins	Mrs. Lambert N.	1583	01-Jun-1848	F	fifth child
Hopkins	Mrs. Lambert N.	2128	02-Apr-1852	M	
Hopkins	Mrs. M. A.	2624	22-Jul-1855	F	first child
Hopkins	Mrs. M. A.	2965	18-Sep-1857	M	second child
Hopkins	Mrs. Seth	4821	09-Mar-1873	M	second pregnancy
Hopkins	Mrs. Wm. C.	3312	26-Dec-1859	F	third child
Hopkins	Mrs. Wm. S.	3822	25-Nov-1863		fourth pregnancy

Obstetrical Casebooks of Dr. F. E. Chatard – an alternative genealogical resource 1829-1883

Hopper	Mrs. D. W.	4895	04-Apr-1874	M	first pregnancy
Horwitz	Mrs. Orville	3847	24-Jan-1864		second pregnancy, "Her father, Dr. Gross of Philadelphia officiated … she had a long and tedious convalescence."
Horwitz	Mrs. Theophilus	3557	22-Aug-1861	F	first child. "She had considerable hemorrhage after birth of child & was very feeble for many hours."
Hosmer	Mrs. James R.	3322	10-Jan-1860	F	first child
Houck	Mrs. A.	3030	02-Jan-1858	F	seventh child
Houck	Mrs. A. V.	1417	04-Apr-1847	F	second child
Houck	Mrs. A. V.	1726	17-Jul-1849	F	third child
Houck	Mrs. A. V.	2025	05-Sep-1851	M	fourth child
Houck	Mrs. A. V.	2330	08-Sep-1853	M	fifth child
Houck	Mrs. A. V.	2636	16-Aug-1855	M	sixth child
Houck	Mrs. A. V>	3377	29-May-1860	M	eighth child
Houck	Mrs. A. V>	3671	23-Aug-1862	F/F	eighth child
Houck	Mrs. Anthony	1112	28-Jan-1845	F	first child
Houck	Mrs. Frederick	1632	15-Oct-1848	F	third child
Houck	Mrs. Theodore	3561	25-Aug-1861	F	first child
Hough	Mrs.	329	24-Aug-1838	M	first child
Hough	Mrs.	493	22-May-1840	F	second child
Hough	Mrs.	991	09-May-1844	M	third child
Hough	Mrs. Robert	4873	29-Dec-1873	F	first pregnancy. "The child, a girl was quite large."
Hough	Mrs. Robert	5043	05-Mar-1876		second pregnancy, forceps delivery
Hough	Mrs. W. D.	5137	13-Jul-1877	M	fourth pregnancy
Houster	Mrs.	82	26-Aug-1833	M	fifth child, nine pounds
Houster	Mrs.	161	22-Oct-1835	F	see 26 Aug 1833 [#82], sixth child
Houster	Mrs. Andrew	2143	02-Jun-1852	M	12th child

98

Obstetrical Casebooks of Dr. F. E. Chatard – an alternative genealogical resource 1829-1883

Houster	Mrs. Andrew	2534	04-Jan-1855	F	13th child
Howard	Mrs.	1454	21-Jul-1847	M	first child
Howard	Mrs. Carrill	702	03-Apr-1842	M	second child
Howard	Mrs. G. W.	776	12-Nov-1842	F	first child
Howard	Mrs. McHenry	4340	12-Jun-1868	F	first pregnancy
Howard	Mrs. McHenry	4542	08-May-1870	M	second pregnancy
Howard	Mrs. McHenry	4890	17-Mar-1874	F	third pregnancy
Howard	Mrs. William R.	5054	13-May-1876	M	second pregnancy
Howard	Mrs. Wm.	4133	11-Aug-1866	M	fifth pregnancy
Howard	Mrs. Wm. Ross	5250	28-Mar-1882	M	fifth pregnancy
Howe	Mrs.	1186	03-Aug-1845	M	second child
Howe	Mrs.	1497	11-Nov-1847	F	third child
Howell	Mrs. R. L.	4237	27-Jul-1867	M	second pregnancy
Hoyt	Mrs. Henry	3491	15-Feb-1861	F	first child
Hoyt	Mrs. Henry	3916	05-Aug-1864	F	second pregnancy
Hubbell	Mrs. E.	2679	16-Nov-1855	F	first child
Hubbell	Mrs. Eben.	3343	24-Feb-1860	M	fourth child
Huggins	Mrs.	834	15-Mar-1843	F	first child, stillborn
Huggins	Mrs. Josiah	1464	12-Aug-1847	M	fourth child
Hughes	Mrs.	71	16-Apr-1833	M	second child
Hughes	Mrs. Felix	209	01-Oct-1836	F	fourth child
Hughes	Mrs. George	548	26-Nov-1840	M	first child, forceps delivery, stillborn
Hughes	Mrs. George	805	07-Jan-1843	F	second child
Hughes	Mrs. George	1174	06-Jul-1845	F	second child
Hughes	Mrs. James	4930	06-Sep-1874	F	second pregnancy, 11 pounds
Hughes	Mrs. John	2659	26-Sep-1855	F	first child

Obstetrical Casebooks of Dr. F. E. Chatard – an alternative genealogical resource 1829-1883

Hughes	Mrs. N. B.	1213	05-Oct-1845	F	second child
Hughes	Mrs. W. J. S.	5114	03-Apr-1877	M	second pregnancy
Hughes	Mrs. William J. S.	5035	24-Jan-1876	M	first pregnancy
Huisler	Mrs. Charles	1537	30-Jan-1848	F	second child
Hungerford	Mrs.	336	15-Sep-1838	M	first child
Hunichenn	Mrs.	979	31-Mar-1844	M	second child
Hunichenn	Mrs.	1155	21-May-1845	F	third child
Hunichenn	Mrs.	1633	18-Oct-1848	M	fifth child
Hunicken	Mrs.	700	29-Mar-1842	F	first child
Hunnichenn	Mrs.	1374	02-Jan-1847	M	fourth child
Huntenwaller	Mrs.	1314	07-Aug-1846	M	seventh child
Hunter	Mrs.	340	11-Oct-1838		first child
Hunter	Mrs. Adam	2207	17-Nov-1852	M	first child
Hunter	Mrs. Adam	2896	05-May-1857	M	second child
Hunter	Mrs. Henry	3922	11-Sep-1864	F	second pregnancy
Huntermuller	Mrs.	1474	06-Sep-1847	M	ninth child, difficult birth, child dead
Hurlbut	Mrs. Samuel	1923	01-Dec-1850	M	second child
Hurst	Mrs. W. R.	3602	30-Dec-1861	F	third child
Husband	Mrs. J. J.	2521	06-Dec-1854	F	third child
Huster	Mrs. W. W.	4418	08-Feb-1869	F	sixth pregnancy
Hustis	Mrs. Andrew	4006	19-May-1865	F	third pregnancy
Hutchins	Mrs. Sarah	2479	15-Sep-1854	F	first child
Hutchins	Mrs. Sarah	2743	29-Apr-1856	M	second child
Hutchins	Mrs. Thomas	3089	31-May-1858		third child

Obstetrical Casebooks of Dr. F. E. Chatard – an alternative genealogical resource 1829-1883

Hutchinson	Mrs. E. S.	3530	09-Jun-1861	F	second child
Hutchinson	Mrs. E. S.	3690	15-Oct-1862	M	third child
Hutchinson	Mrs. E. S.	3919	30-Aug-1864	M	fourth pregnancy
Hutchinson	Mrs. E. S.	4168	16-Dec-1866	F	fifth pregnancy
Hutter	Mrs. Henry	3472	28-Dec-1860	F	first child
Hutton	Mrs. Henry	4201	07-Mar-1867	F	third pregnancy
Hutton	Mrs. N. H.	4013	07-Jun-1865		second pregnancy
Hyatt	Mrs. Edward	3245	01-Jun-1859	M	first child
Hyatt	Mrs. Edward	3895	01-Jun-1864	F	second pregnancy
Hyatt	Mrs. Edward	3895	01-Jun-1864	F	second pregnancy
Hyde	Mrs. Arnold	4289	18-Dec-1867	M	first pregnancy, "It was a boy but gave no sign of life."
Hyde	Mrs. Arnold	4409	22-Jan-1869	M	second pregnancy
Hyde	Mrs. Arnold	4695	01-Oct-1871	F	second pregnancy, seven months, "The child gave no signs of life. It was deformed having a hare lip, dilated feet & a tumor projecting from the occiput."
Hyde	Mrs. E.	325	17-Aug-1838	M	first child
Hyde	Mrs. Moses	395	10-Jul-1839	M	first child
Hyde	Mrs. Moses	624	13-Aug-1841	M	second child
Hyde	Mrs. Moses	780	19-Nov-1842	F	third child
Hyde	Mrs. Moses	1421	12-Apr-1847	M	fifth child
Hyde	Mrs. Moses	1652	04-Dec-1848	M	sixth child
Hyde	Mrs. Moses	1913	11-Nov-1850	M	seventh child
Hyde	Mrs. Moses	2138	25-May-1852	M	eighth child
Hyde	Mrs. Moses	3108	01-Aug-1853	F	ninth child
Hysan	Mrs. Wm.	4840	18-Jun-1873	F	seventh pregnancy. "All her labours have been difficult and the forceps

Obstetrical Casebooks of Dr. F. E. Chatard – an alternative genealogical resource 1829-1883

Hyson	Mrs. William	4475	07-Aug-1869	F	had been used in every case."
Ingle	Mrs. W. P.	3120	27-Aug-1858	M	fifth pregnancy, forceps delivery
Ingle	Mrs. Wm.	3523	17-May-1861	M	first child
Ingle	Mrs. Wm.	3682	23-Sep-1862	M	second child
Iniford	Mrs. Joseph	2979	10-Oct-1857	M	third child
Inimer	Mrs.	39	03-Jan-1832		eight child, attended by midwife, "She [mother] was extremely impatient … the child, a fine and stout one gave no signs of life & all attempts to make it breath proved abortive
Inloes	Mrs. J. S.	580	20-Mar-1841	F	eighth child
Ireland	Mrs. Samuel L.	4829	26-Apr-1873	M	third pregnancy
Irving	Mrs. T.	3391	01-Jul-1860	F	second child
Irving	Mrs. Thomas	3116	24-Aug-1858	M	first child
Irving	Mrs. Thomas	4449	16-May-1869	M	fourth pregnancy
Irving	Mrs. Thomas	3636	11-May-1862	M	third child
Israel	Mrs. William	279	03-Feb-1838	F	first child
J. W.	Miss	1210	02-Oct-1845	M	first child
Jackson	Mary	1436	21-May-1847	M	colored, fifth child
Jackson	Mary	2580	07-Apr-1855	F	colored, 10th child
Jackson	Mrs.	130	29-Dec-1834	M	colored, first child, six months, child died
Jackson	Mrs.	197	05-Aug-1836	M	colored, second child
Jackson	Mrs. Willis	295	03-Apr-1838	F	third child
Jackson	Mrs. Willis	982	08-Apr-1844	M	colored, third child
Jackson	Mrs. Willis	1217	20-Oct-1845	F	colored, fourth child
Jackson	Mrs. Willis	1599	08-Jul-1848	F	colored, eighth month
Jackson	Mrs. Willis	1956	02-Mar-1851	M	colored, premature 5 months

Obstetrical Casebooks of Dr. F. E. Chatard – an alternative genealogical resource 1829-1883

Jackson	Mrs. Willis	2317	06-Aug-1853	F	colored, ninth child
Jacobsen	Mrs.	105	25-May-1834	M	ninth child, 7 3/4 pounds
Jamaies	Mrs. Dr. W. D.	2054	11-Nov-1851	F	third child
Jamart	Mrs. Lewis	2957	03-Sep-1857	M	third child
Jamart	Mrs. Louis	2321	14-Aug-1853	F	first child
Jamart	Mrs. Louis	3251	02-Jul-1859	F	fourth child
Jamart	Mrs. Louis	3555	13-Aug-1861	F	fifth child
Jamart	Mrs. Louis	3842	14-Jan-1864	F	sixth pregnancy
Jamart	Mrs. Louis A.	2633	12-Aug-1855	M	second child
James	Mrs. Henry	4960	05-Dec-1874	F	fourth pregnancy, eight months, child dead
James	Susan	2690	17-Dec-1855	F/F	colored, first child, eighth month, twins
James	Susan	2940	22-Jul-1857	M	second child
James	Susan	3314	28-Dec-1859	M	colored, fourth child
James	Susan	3685	26-Sep-1862	F	colored, fifth child
Jamet	Mrs. Edward	5149	26-Sep-1877	F	first pregnancy
Jamet	Mrs. Edward	5205	27-Oct-1879	M	second pregnancy
Jamieson	Mrs. Andrew	4096	27-Mar-1866	M	first pregnancy
Jamieson	Mrs. Dr. W. D.	4179	24-Jan-1867	M	eighth pregnancy
Janes	Mrs. Henry	5023	17-Dec-1875	M	fourth pregnancy, 7.5 months
Janes [Jones]	Mrs. H.	1947	10-Feb-1851	M	premature 7 months, stillborn
Jeanneret	Mrs.	3845	16-Jan-1864	F	first pregnancy
Jeannert	Mrs.	4078	25-Jan-1866	F	second pregnancy
Jeannert	Mrs. F.	4317	19-Mar-1868	F	third pregnancy
Jeannert	Mrs. J. P.	4164	05-Dec-1866	M	first pregnancy
Jeannert	Mrs. L.	4454	21-May-1869	M	fourth pregnancy
Jeannert	Mrs. L.	4679	19-Jul-1871	M	fifth pregnancy

Obstetrical Casebooks of Dr. F. E. Chatard – an alternative genealogical resource 1829-1883

Jeannert	Mrs. L. P.	4314	14-Mar-1868	F	second pregnancy
Jeannert	Mrs. L. P.	4540	03-May-1870	F	third pregnancy
Jeans	Mrs. Henry	4343	16-Jun-1868	M	first pregnancy
Jenkins	Mrs. Alfred	829	08-Mar-1843	F	third child
Jenkins	Mrs. Alfred	1063	24-Oct-1844	M	born 9:30 AM
Jenkins	Mrs. Anthony	2171	02-Sep-1852	M	fifth child
Jenkins	Mrs. Anthony	2537	07-Jan-1855	M	fourth child
Jenkins	Mrs. Anthony	3100	20-Jul-1858	F	fifth child
Jenkins	Mrs. Anthony H.	1379	18-Jan-1847	F	second child
Jenkins	Mrs. Arthur	620	11-Aug-1841	M	first child
Jenkins	Mrs. Austin	1045	04-Oct-1844	F	second child
Jenkins	Mrs. Austin	1297	25-Jun-1846	F	second child
Jenkins	Mrs. Austin	1594	30-Jun-1848	M	fourth child
Jenkins	Mrs. Austin	2026	08-Sep-1851	F	born about 8 PM
Jenkins	Mrs. Austin	2287	27-May-1853	M	sixth child
Jenkins	Mrs. Austin	2621	18-Jul-1855	M	seventh child
Jenkins	Mrs. Austin	2862	18-Feb-1857	M	eighth child
Jenkins	Mrs. Burton	3021	18-Dec-1857	F	attended by Dr G. Gibson
Jenkins	Mrs. Courtney	550	27-Nov-1840	F	
Jenkins	Mrs. Courtney	1299	28-Jun-1846	F	sixth child
Jenkins	Mrs. Courtney	1745	11-Sep-1849	M	eighth child
Jenkins	Mrs. Edward	1795	12-Jan-1850	F	first child, It was in a state of asphyxia & was recalled to life with great difficulty.
Jenkins	Mrs. Edward	1954	01-Mar-1851	F	second child

Obstetrical Casebooks of Dr. F. E. Chatard – an alternative genealogical resource 1829-1883

Jenkins	Mrs. Edward	2204	14-Nov-1852	M	third child
Jenkins	Mrs. Edward	2412	16-Apr-1854	M	fourth child
Jenkins	Mrs. Edward	2710	07-Feb-1856	F	fourth child
Jenkins	Mrs. Edward	2962	13-Sep-1857	F	fifth child
Jenkins	Mrs. Edward	3594	27-Nov-1861	M	seventh child
Jenkins	Mrs. F. X.	4766	15-Jul-1872	M	first pregnancy
Jenkins	Mrs. G. C.	4920	18-Aug-1874	F	third pregnancy
Jenkins	Mrs. G. T.	3200	23-Feb-1859	M	fifth child
Jenkins	Mrs. George C.	4777	07-Sep-1872	F	second pregnancy
Jenkins	Mrs. George T.	1914	12-Nov-1850	F	first child
Jenkins	Mrs. George T.	2034	09-Oct-1851	F	second child
Jenkins	Mrs. George T.	2302	07-Jul-1853	M	third child
Jenkins	Mrs. George T.	2483	21-Sep-1854	F	fourth child
Jenkins	Mrs. Hugh	591	30-Apr-1841	M	first child
Jenkins	Mrs. Hugh	925	29-Nov-1843	M	second child
Jenkins	Mrs. J. W.	725	15-Jun-1842	M	second child
Jenkins	Mrs. James	327	20-Aug-1838	M	fourth child
Jenkins	Mrs. James	535	19-Oct-1840	M	
Jenkins	Mrs. James	890	13-Sep-1843	M	born 1 AM
Jenkins	Mrs. James	1164	08-Jun-1845	F	born about 1 PM
Jenkins	Mrs. James	1410	27-Mar-1847	M	eight child
Jenkins	Mrs. Joseph	964	27-Feb-1844	M	third child, he died the next day
Jenkins	Mrs. Joseph	1393	09-Feb-1847	F	fifth child
Jenkins	Mrs. Joseph	3076	26-Apr-1858	M	second child
Jenkins	Mrs. Joseph	3531	10-Jun-1861	M	fourth child

Obstetrical Casebooks of Dr. F. E. Chatard – an alternative genealogical resource 1829-1883

Jenkins	Mrs. Joseph W.	598	31-May-1841	M	first child
Jenkins	Mrs. Joseph W.	1664	21-Jan-1849	M	sixth child, mother died on 29th
Jenkins	Mrs. Joseph W.	2839	11-Dec-1856	M	first child, died
Jenkins	Mrs. Joseph W.	3258	25-Jul-1859	M	third child
Jenkins	Mrs. Joseph W.	3714	14-Dec-1862	M	fifth child
Jenkins	Mrs. Joseph W.	3879	16-Apr-1864	M	sixth pregnancy
Jenkins	Mrs. Robert	1533	19-Jan-1848	M	second child
Jenkins	Mrs. Robert J.	1318	15-Aug-1846	M	first child
Jenkins	Mrs. T. P.	1358	26-Nov-1846	F	second child
Jenkins	Mrs. T. Robert	1884	08-Sep-1850	M	third child
Jenkins	Mrs. Thomas	1231	26-Nov-1845	M	first child
Jenkins	Mrs. Thomas W.	4065	24-Dec-1865	F	second pregnancy
Jenkins	Mrs. Thomas W.	4246	29-Aug-1867	M	third pregnancy
Jenkins	Mrs. Thomas W.	4435	26-Mar-1869	F	fourth pregnancy
Jenkins	Mrs. Thomas W.	4719	10-Dec-1871	M	fifth pregnancy
Jenkins	Mrs. Thomas W.	4865	10-Nov-1873	M	sixth pregnancy
Jenkins	Mrs. Thomas W.	4995	04-Aug-1875	M	seventh child
Jenkins	Mrs. Thomas W.	5128	18-Jun-1877	M	eighth pregnancy, stillborn. "Some hours before the labor commenced, she had a fainting spell & complained of a very tight feeling about the womb."

Obstetrical Casebooks of Dr. F. E. Chatard – an alternative genealogical resource 1829-1883

Jenkins	Mrs. Thornton	1768	27-Oct-1849	F	first child
Jenkins	Mrs. Thornton	2194	24-Oct-1852	M	second child
Jenkins	Mrs. Thornton	2509	11-Nov-1854	M	third child
Jenkins	Mrs. Thorton	3532	12-Jun-1861	F	fifth child, eight months
Jenkins, Jr.	Mrs. Austin	4801	07-Dec-1872	M	third pregnancy
Jenkins, Jr.	Mrs. Joseph W.	4594	03-Oct-1870	M	second pregnancy
Jenkins, Jr.	Mrs. Joseph W.	4728	31-Dec-1871	F	third pregnancy, forceps delivery
Jenkins, Jr.	Mrs. Joseph W.	5026	25-Dec-1875	M/	fourth pregnancy, eight months, twins. "She gave birth to twins during her first confinement."
Jenkins, Jr.	Mrs. Thomas C.	2932	07-Jul-1857	M	first child, "She had not felt the child for about six weeks." It was dead
Johnson	Miss Caroline	2249	24-Feb-1853	M	mother and child died
Johnson	Mrs.	3302	07-Dec-1859	F	at St. Vincent's Asylum, third child
Johnson	Mrs. Dr. C.	2837	08-Dec-1856	M	first child
Johnson	Mrs. Dr. C.	3092	05-Jun-1858	M	second child
Johnson	Mrs. E. C.	4589	23-Sep-1870	F	first pregnancy, premature at eight months but healthy
Johnson	Mrs. Edward	4680	21-Jul-1871	F	second pregnancy
Johnson	Mrs. Edward	4764	02-Jul-1872	M	first pregnancy, "A case of prolonged gestation."
Johnson	Mrs. J. M.	4283	23-Nov-1867	M	first pregnancy, attended by Dr. Cathell
Johnson	Mrs. James	2175	07-Sep-1852	M	second child
Johnson	Mrs. Josiah L.	3611	31-Jan-1862	F	first child
Johnson	Mrs. S. M.	3886	09-May-1864	F	third pregnancy
Johnson	Mrs. Thomas M.	3013	03-Dec-1857	F	fourth child
Johnston	Mrs. Dr. Ch.	4376	11-Oct-1868		ninth pregnancy, in labour about 41 hours, child died
Johnston	Mrs. Henry E.	4159	21-Nov-1866	M	first pregnancy

107

Obstetrical Casebooks of Dr. F. E. Chatard – an alternative genealogical resource 1829-1883

Johnston	Mrs. Henry E.	4534	24-Mar-1870	M	second pregnancy, forceps delivery
Jones	Emily	651	29-Oct-1841	F	colored, second child
Jones	Emily	1016	27-Jul-1844	F	colored, third child
Jones	Mrs.	125	01-Dec-1834	F	first child
Jones	Mrs. Alonzo V.	2048	29-Oct-1851	F	first child, died a few hours after birth
Jones	Mrs. Catherine	1461	04-Aug-1847	M	first child
Jones	Mrs. Catherine	1929	19-Dec-1850	M	third child
Jones	Mrs. G. F.	3250	21-Jun-1859	M	first child
Jones	Mrs. Isaiah	950	21-Jan-1844	M	second child
Jones	Mrs. J. H.	3860	01-Mar-1864	F	second pregnancy. "This patient was attacked with hemiplegia about two weeks previous to confinement. The paralytic affection was not much relieved by the birth
Jones	Mrs. J. N.	746	16-Aug-1842	F	first child
Jones	Mrs. John	826	01-Mar-1843	M	colored, first child
Jones	Mrs. John R.	3473	30-Dec-1860	M	first child
Jones, Jr.	Mrs. Samuel	935	19-Dec-1843	M	sixth child
Jordan	Mrs. Charles	4822	21-Mar-1873	M	second pregnancy, "This patient was so nervous & screamed so loud that I was nervous & screamed so loud that I was obliged to give her chloroform."
Jordan	Mrs. Charles	4997	22-Aug-1875	F	third pregnancy
Jordon	Mrs. C.	4701	25-Oct-1871	F	first pregnancy, forceps delivery
Judge	Mrs. Henry	728	26-Jun-1842	M	second child
Justis	Mrs. W.	175	04-Jan-1836	M	first child
K.	Miss	3137	01-Oct-1858	F	first child
Kaefold	Mrs. Charles J.	2029	03-Oct-1851	F	first child
Kahler	Mrs. Charles	4712	30-Nov-1871	F	second pregnancy

Obstetrical Casebooks of Dr. F. E. Chatard – an alternative genealogical resource 1829-1883

Surname	Name	Case #	Date	Sex	Notes
Kahler	Mrs. Charles	4904	25-May-1874	F	third pregnancy
Kahler	Mrs. Charles	5012	16-Oct-1875	F	fourth pregnancy. "She complained greatly during & previous to her confinement of intense headache and diminished urine. On examining her urine I found that she was labouring under diabetes insipidus."
Kamp	Mrs. John	3512	28-Apr-1861	M	first child
Kane	Mrs. Darby	2658	22-Sep-1855	M	first child
Kane	Mrs. James	4386	18-Nov-1868	M	first pregnancy, "The child presented a formidable hairlip inclining the head & soft palate to the left side. A child by a prior marriage … about 6 years old is affected with similar manner."
Kane	Mrs. Wm. Darby	2925	25-Jun-1857	F	see 22 Sep 1855, third child. "At her urgent demand, I applied the forceps and extracted the child."
Karr	Mrs. Nicholas	1759	06-Oct-1849	M	first child
Katz	Mrs.	1433	16-May-1847	M	second child
Katz	Mrs.	2153	07-Jul-1852	M	fourth child
Katz	Mrs.	2340	03-Oct-1853	M	fifth child
Katz	Mrs. J.	1264	02-Mar-1846	M	first child
Katz	Mrs. J.	2533	29-Dec-1854	M	sixth child
Katz	Mrs. John	1910	07-Nov-1850	F	third child
Keach	Mrs. P. H.	1179	14-Jul-1845		first child
Kealy	Mrs. John D.	4470	26-Jul-1869	M	first pregnancy
Keedy	Mrs. Dr.	4207	16-Apr-1867	F	first pregnancy
Keenahan	Mrs. Barclay	2998	13-Nov-1857	M	first child
Keenan	Mrs. D.	4452	18-May-1869	M	third pregnancy
Keenan	Mrs. D.	4631	06-Jan-1871	M	fourth pregnancy
Keenan	Mrs. Daniel	4209	19-Apr-1867	M	second pregnancy
Keenan	Mrs. Daniel	4793	02-Nov-1872	F	fifth pregnancy

Obstetrical Casebooks of Dr. F. E. Chatard – an alternative genealogical resource 1829-1883

Keenan	Mrs. Daniel	4947	01-Nov-1874	M	sixth pregnancy
Keenan	Mrs. J.	0	03-Nov-1848		first child, attended by midwife, complications
Keenan	Mrs. Joseph	3607	22-Jan-1862	M	second child
Keer	Mrs. C. G.	4301	31-Jan-1868	F	first pregnancy
Keer	Mrs. Charles G.	4520	01-Jan-1870	F	second pregnancy
Keer	Mrs. Charles G.	5039	04-Feb-1876	M	third pregnancy
Keerl	Mrs. Henry	1059	20-Oct-1844	F	second child
Kees	Mrs.	632	18-Sep-1841	F	child born when MD arrived
Kees	Mrs. Peter	152	25-Jul-1835	M	"This lady is of a very delicate health"
Kees	Mrs. Peter	230	11-Apr-1837	F	born in half an hour
Keghler	Mrs. John	4083	19-Feb-1866	M	first pregnancy
Keighler	Mrs.	1283	22-May-1846	M	born 4:20 PM
Keighler	Mrs. W.	672	16-Jan-1842	M	fourth child
Keighler	Mrs. William	1552	13-Mar-1848	M	born 3 PM
Keighler	Mrs. William	1791	25-Dec-1849	F	eighth child
Keighler	Mrs. Wm.	955	04-Feb-1844	F	fifth child
Keiholtz	Mrs. Otis	3862	02-Mar-1864	F	second pregnancy
Keiholtz	Mrs. Otis	4073	18-Jan-1866	F	third pregnancy
Keilholtz	Mrs. Otis	3629	22-Apr-1862	M	first child
Keilholtz	Mrs. Otis	4363	10-Aug-1868	M	fourth pregnancy
Keirl	Mrs. Wm.	540	04-Nov-1840	M	first child
Keirnan	Mrs. J.	1874	06-Aug-1850	F	second child
Keith	Mrs. William	4724	25-Dec-1871	M	second pregnancy, 7 1/2 months. "He cried strongly & appeared to breath freely, it soon however began to moan & died the next morning."
Kelly	Mrs.	1459	03-Aug-1847	F	mother died on 6th August from lacerated uterus

Obstetrical Casebooks of Dr. F. E. Chatard – an alternative genealogical resource 1829-1883

Kelly	Mrs. Alexander	1032	31-Aug-1844	M	second child, stillborn
Kelly	Mrs. Alexander	1139	06-Apr-1845	M	premature, four months
Kelly	Mrs. J. J.	5111	26-Mar-1877	F	second pregnancy
Kelly	Mrs. J. J.	5174	21-Nov-1878	M	third pregnancy, forceps delivery
Kelly	Mrs. J. J.	5220	23-Jun-1880	F	fourth pregnancy
Kelly	Mrs. J. W.	3970	09-Jan-1865	F	seventh pregnancy, stillborn
Kelly	Mrs. James	2130	30-Apr-1852	F	second child
Kelly	Mrs. John	4163	03-Dec-1866	F	seventh pregnancy
Kelly	Mrs. John J.	5254	21-Apr-1882	M	fifth pregnancy, forceps delivery. Weight 13.5 lbs
Kelly	Mrs. Mcl.	1682	26-Feb-1849	M	attended by Dr. C. Johnson
Kelly	Mrs. Patrick	1967	03-Apr-1851	M	second child
Kelly	Mrs. Patrick	2236	31-Jan-1853	M	third child
Kelly	Mrs. Patrick	2411	14-Apr-1854	M	first child
Kelly	Mrs. Patrick	2610	28-Jun-1855	F	second child
Kelly	Mrs. Patrick	3039	01-Feb-1858	M	fourth child
Kelly	Mrs. Terence	2489	29-Sep-1854	F	fourth child
Kelly	Mrs. William	4072	17-Jan-1866	F	third pregnancy
Kelly	Mrs. Wm.	3912	27-Jul-1864	M	second pregnancy. "I left her in care of a midwife."
Kelly, Jr.	Mrs. A.	918	11-Nov-1843		premature labor, four months
Kemp	Mrs. E.	622	12-Aug-1841	F	fifth child
Kemp	Mrs. E. D.	286	01-Mar-1838	F	third child
Kemp	Mrs. R.	3820	14-Nov-1863		third pregnancy
Kemp	Mrs. R. C.	4144	04-Sep-1866	M	fourth pregnancy
Kemp	Mrs. R. C.	4726	27-Dec-1871	F	sixth pregnancy
Kemp	Mrs. R. C.	4864	27-Oct-1873	F	seventh pregnancy

111

Obstetrical Casebooks of Dr. F. E. Chatard – an alternative genealogical resource 1829-1883

Kemp	Mrs. R. C.	5069	19-Jul-1876	M	eighth pregnancy
Kemp	Mrs. R.C.	3447	26-Nov-1860	F	second child
Kemp	Mrs. Richard C.	3090	01-Jun-1858	M	first child
Kemp	Mrs. Thomas	4489	05-Oct-1869	M	tenth pregnancy, "affected with spina bifida & both feet deformed." child died
Kemp	Mrs. Thomas	4636	17-Jan-1871	F	12th pregnancy
Kempton	Mrs.	347	05-Nov-1838	F	first child
Kendall	Mrs. Wm. J.	3508	16-Apr-1861	F	second child
Kenley	Mrs.	1755	28-Sep-1849	F	third child
Kennard	Mrs. George	404	05-Aug-1839	F	first child
Kennard	Mrs. George J.	621	11-Aug-1841	F	second child
Kennedy	Mrs. James	2309	23-Jul-1853	M	sixth child
Kennedy	Mrs. James P.	978	29-Mar-1844	M	third child
Kennedy	Mrs. James P.	1280	11-May-1846	F	third child
Kennedy	Mrs. James P.	1698	02-Apr-1849	F	fifth child
Kennedy	Mrs. James P.	1986	11-Jun-1851	F	sixth child
Kennedy	Mrs. James P.	2654	11-Sep-1855	F	eighth child
Kennedy	Mrs. James P.	2949	19-Aug-1857	F	ninth child
Kennedy	Mrs. James P.	3328	21-Jan-1860	F	tenth child
Kennedy	Mrs. John	4104	21-May-1866	F	first pregnancy
Kennedy	Mrs. John	4291	23-Dec-1867	M	second pregnancy
Kennedy	Mrs. John	4600	23-Oct-1870	F	third pregnancy
Kennedy	Mrs. Michael	998	08-Jun-1844	M	born 20 minutes before 11 PM
Keney	Mrs.	719	22-May-1842	M	first child
Keney	Mrs. Edwards	4928	31-Aug-1874	F	first pregnancy, forceps delivery
Keney	Mrs. Emily	2549	26-Jan-1855	M	first child

Kenney	Mrs. James	2209	21-Nov-1852	F	first child
Kenny	Mrs. Francis	3893	30-May-1864	M	second pregnancy
Kenny	Mrs. Frank	3753	28-Feb-1863	M	first pregnancy
Kerchner	Mrs. F. A.	2582	09-Apr-1855	F	first child
Kerchoff	Mrs. G.	3831	24-Dec-1863	F	sixth pregnancy
Kerckhoff	Mrs. G.	4287	09-Dec-1867	F	eighth pregnancy
Kerckoff	Mrs. G.	4088	28-Feb-1866	F	seventh pregnancy
Kernan	Mrs.	85	10-Oct-1833		an abortion of about six weeks
Kernan	Mrs. Edward	2220	17-Dec-1852	M	first child
Kernan	Mrs. Michael	1877	16-Aug-1850	M	first child
Kernan	Mrs. P.	119	27-Sep-1834	F	see 10 Oct 1833 [#85], first child
Kernan	Mrs. P.	194	28-Jul-1836		abortion of about six weeks
Kernan	Mrs. P.	256	12-Sep-1837	M	second child
Kernan	Mrs. Peter	492	15-May-1840	F	third child
Kernan	Mrs. Peter	749	24-Aug-1842	F	fourth child
Kernan	Mrs. Peter	1249	14-Jan-1846	F	sixth child
Kernan	Mrs. Peter	1613	12-Aug-1848	F	born a little after 12 midnight
Kernan	Mrs. Peter	1857	30-Jun-1850	M	eighth child
Kernan	Mrs. Peter	2626	01-Aug-1855	M	eighth child
Kernan	Mrs. W.	1449	02-Jul-1847	M	born 9:15 AM
Kerr	Mrs.	28	08-Oct-1831	M	first child, eight pounds
Kessler	Mrs. Samuel	4391	30-Nov-1868	F	third pregnancy
Kessler	Mrs. Sl.	4266	22-Oct-1867	F	first pregnancy
Key	Mrs. Barton	1614	18-Aug-1848	F	third child
Key	Mrs. Barton	1883	02-Sep-1850	F	fourth child

Obstetrical Casebooks of Dr. F. E. Chatard – an alternative genealogical resource 1829-1883

Keys	Mrs. Joseph	4185	02-Feb-1867	M	sixth pregnancy
Keyser	Mrs. M. F.	2059	16-Nov-1851	F	second child
Keyser	Mrs. M. T.	2217	09-Dec-1852	M	third child
Kielly	Mrs. Edward	1383	25-Jan-1847	F	third child, Born before I arrived
Kiersted	Mrs. A. J.	4174	10-Jan-1867	M	first pregnancy
Kimpton	Mrs. W.	129	16-Dec-1834	F	first child, "The umbilical cord did not separate from the child until the nineteenth day."
King	Mrs. George	4932	13-Sep-1874	F	first pregnancy
King	Mrs. Jacob	1423	18-Apr-1847	F	born about 6 AM
King	Mrs. John	4356	25-Jul-1868	M	first pregnancy
King	Mrs. Nicholas	458	27-Jan-1840	F	second child
King	Mrs. Nicholas	691	05-Mar-1842	F	third child
King	Mrs. Nicholas	1629	10-Oct-1848	F	third child
King	Mrs. Wallace	3719	19-Dec-1862	M	first child
King	Mrs. Wallace	4057	01-Dec-1865	M	second pregnancy
King	Mrs. Wallace	4773	27-Aug-1872	M	first pregnancy
King	Mrs. Wallace	4856	24-Sep-1873	F	second pregnancy
King, Jr.	Mrs. John	3051	06-Mar-1858	F	first child
Kinsley	Mrs. S. G.	4380	25-Oct-1868	M	second pregnancy, eight months
Kinsley	Mrs. Saml.	4555	27-May-1870	M	third pregnancy
Kirby	Mrs. Dennis	2882	18-Mar-1857	M	second child
Kirby	Mrs. Dennis	2655	15-Sep-1855	F	first child
Kirby	Mrs. Dennis	3164	18-Nov-1858	M	third child
Kirby	Mrs. Dennis	3513	30-Apr-1861	F	fourth child
Kirby	Mrs. Dennis	3750	21-Feb-1863	M	fifth pregnancy
Kirby	Mrs. Dennis	3989	06-Apr-1865	F	sixth pregnancy

Obstetrical Casebooks of Dr. F. E. Chatard – an alternative genealogical resource 1829-1883

Kirby	Mrs. George A.	4970	17-Jan-1875	F	first pregnancy
Kirby	Mrs. Joseph	4969	08-Jan-1875	M	second pregnancy
Kirkland	Mrs. E. M.	4477	08-Aug-1869	F	first pregnancy
Kirkland	Mrs. E. M.	4612	02-Dec-1870	M	second pregnancy
Kirkland	Mrs. Edward	5099	24-Jan-1877	F	third pregnancy
Kirkland	Mrs. O. A.	5046	29-Mar-1876	F	first pregnancy
Kirkland	Mrs. O. A.	5159	06-Jun-1878	F	third pregnancy
Kirkland	Mrs. O. A.	5264	19-Apr-1883	F	fifth pregnancy
Kirkland	Mrs. Ogden	5113	31-Mar-1877	M	second pregnancy
Kirkland	Mrs. Ogden	5201	14-Sep-1879	F	fourth pregnancy
Kirkland	Mrs. R. R.	1961	10-Mar-1851	M	born 4:15 AM
Kirkley	Mrs.	2934	09-Jul-1857	M	seventh child
Kitty	Mrs. C. J.	4819	07-Mar-1873	F	third pregnancy
Kleckgether	Mrs. D.	4123	27-Jul-1866	M	first pregnancy. "… at rather a mature age… she was confined about 7 o'clock and died the following night."
Klunk	Mrs. C.	4684	02-Aug-1871	M	third pregnancy
Klunk	Mrs. C. S.	4567	25-Jun-1870	M	second pregnancy
Knir [?]	Mrs. J.	3358	01-Apr-1860	F	first child, attended by Dr. Inloes
Knorer	Mrs. E. C.	4557	30-May-1870	M	second pregnancy
Knorer	Mrs. Edward	4359	05-Aug-1868	M	first pregnancy
Knox	Mrs. Fay	5021	03-Dec-1875	F	second pregnancy
Knox	Mrs. James	3569	12-Sep-1861	M	second child
Knox	Mrs. James	3728	02-Jan-1863	F	third child
Knox	Mrs. W. Fay	4906	06-Jun-1874	F	first pregnancy
Kohn	Mrs. N.	4916	22-Jul-1874	F	third pregnancy, ninth month, hemorrhaging, child dead
Kolfold	Mrs. Charles J.	2430	29-May-1854	M	second child

115

Obstetrical Casebooks of Dr. F. E. Chatard – an alternative genealogical resource 1829-1883

Kosier	Mrs.	273	23-Dec-1837	F	second child
Kosier	Mrs.	408	13-Aug-1839	F	third child
Kraft	Mrs. W.	4807	18-Dec-1872	M	first pregnancy
Kratz	Mrs. J. Nicholas	1903	24-Oct-1850	F	seventh child
Krauth	Mrs. C. P.	1206	21-Sep-1845	F	first child
Kreamer	Mrs.	188	18-May-1836	F	first child
Kreamer	Mrs. James	1561	17-Apr-1848	F	eighth child
Kreamer	Mrs. James	2524	12-Dec-1854	F	11th child
Kreamer	Mrs. John	3709	01-Dec-1862	F	second child
Kremelberg	Mrs. J.	3811	24-Sep-1863	M	first pregnancy
Kremelberg	Mrs. J. D.	4528	22-Feb-1870	F	fourth pregnancy
Kremer	Mrs.	308	27-Jun-1838	F	second child
Kremer	Mrs.	536	21-Oct-1840	M	third child
Kremer	Mrs.	757	06-Sep-1842	F	fourth child
Kremer	Mrs. J.	948	19-Jan-1844	F	fourth child
Kremer	Mrs. Jacob	499	15-Jun-1840	M	first child
Kremer	Mrs. James	1276	01-May-1846	F	The child was born when I arrived
Kremer	Mrs. James	1744	09-Sep-1849	F	ninth child
Kremer	Mrs. James	2102	17-Feb-1852	M	tenth child
Kugler	Mrs. B.	1635	20-Oct-1848	F	fifth child
L.	Miss	3409	25-Aug-1860	M	at St. Vincent's Asylum, first child
Lacey	Mrs. James	3653	01-Jul-1862	F	first child
Lacy	Mrs. Maurice	3931	02-Oct-1864	F	second pregnancy
Ladkin	Mrs. James	2503	25-Oct-1854	F	second child
Ladson	Mrs. W. H.	3135	28-Sep-1858	F	fifth child
Lally	Mrs. Michael	2004	17-Jul-1851	M	first child, attended by Dr. Patterson

116

Obstetrical Casebooks of Dr. F. E. Chatard – an alternative genealogical resource 1829-1883

Lambden	Mrs. Thomas	2791	15-Sep-1856	F	first child, expired
Lanaan [?]	Mrs. John	2748	12-May-1856	M	tenth child
Lanahan	Mrs.	469	19-Mar-1840	F	third child
Lanahan	Mrs. J.	4522	06-Jan-1870	F	first pregnancy
Lanahan	Mrs. Wm.	971	20-Mar-1844	M	third child
Lanckoe	Mrs.	223	03-Feb-1837		fourth child, mother with anasarca & ascites, miscarriage
Landsdown	Mrs.	2899	10-May-1857	M	second child, "did not live more than a few hours."
Landstreet	Mrs.	1317	13-Aug-1846	M	second child
Landstreet	Mrs. A. C.	1730	24-Jul-1849	F	third child
Landstreet	Mrs. A. C.	2072	14-Dec-1851	M	fourth child, died
Landstreet	Mrs. A. C.	2359	27-Nov-1853	M	fifth child
Lane	Mrs.	68	11-Mar-1833	M	fourth child
Langdon	Mrs. James	4334	18-May-1863	M	sixth pregnancy
Lanier	Mrs. Lt.	2038	14-Oct-1851	F	first child
Lanier	Mrs. Lucius	4212	25-Apr-1867	F	second pregnancy, "… patient of feeble constitution."
Lanier	Mrs. Lucius L.	4368	31-Aug-1868	M	fourth pregnancy. "She was very delicate & weak."
Lanier	Mrs. Lucius L.	4561	18-Jun-1870	M	fifth pregnancy
Lankford	Mrs.	1193	18-Aug-1845	M	first child, stillborn
Lankie	Mrs. L.	4630	04-Jan-1871	F	second pregnancy
Lannan	Mrs.	648	24-Oct-1841	M	fourth child
Lannan	Mrs.	1304	08-Jul-1846	F	sixth child
Lanner	Mrs.	1657	28-Dec-1848	M	seventh child
Lantz	Mrs.	2252	10-Mar-1853	F	ninth child
Lantz	Mrs. O.	2918	17-Jun-1857	F	first child, stillborn
Lantz	Mrs. Oliver	3139	03-Oct-1858	F	second child

Obstetrical Casebooks of Dr. F. E. Chatard – an alternative genealogical resource 1829-1883

Name		Number	Date	Sex	Notes
Lantz	Mrs. Oliver	3410	29-Aug-1860	F	third child. "The patient had her youth and the pelvis projects inwards on hip disease in the right …" child dead
Lantz	Mrs. Oliver	3758	10-Mar-1863	F	fourth pregnancy
Lantz	Mrs. Oliver	3980	03-Feb-1865	M	fifth pregnancy, forceps delivery, child died. Mother died on 5th.
Lapneraille	Mrs. A.	908	22-Oct-1843	M	second child
Laponaille	Mrs.	1260	13-Feb-1846	F	third child
Larentrie	Mrs. Henry	1868	04-Aug-1850	M	first child
Larkin	Mrs.	553	04-Dec-1840	M/F	twins
Larogue	Mrs. Achille	5118	19-Apr-1877	M	first pregnancy
Larrogue	Mrs. Emile	1812	11-Feb-1850	M	first child
Larrogue	Mrs. Emile	3416	10-Sep-1860	M	seventh child
Larroque	Mrs. Emile	2022	29-Aug-1851	F	second child
Larroque	Mrs. Emile	2276	06-May-1853	M	third child
Larroque	Mrs. Emile	2551	29-Jan-1855	F	fourth child
Larroque	Mrs. Emile	2820	05-Nov-1856	M	fifth child
Larroque	Mrs. Emile	3185	19-Jan-1859	M	sixth child
Larroque	Mrs. Emile	3677	05-Sep-1862	M	eighth child
Latrobe	Mrs. Ferdinand C.	5261	06-Jan-1883	F	fourth pregnancy
Latrobe	Mrs. J.H.B.	1965	23-Mar-1851	F	sixth child
Lattimer	Mrs. G.	2046	25-Oct-1851	M	first child
Laughter	Mrs. W. H.	4674	04-Jul-1871	M	second pregnancy, "the child gave no signs of life."
Laughter	Mrs. Wm. H.	4503	15-Nov-1869	F	first pregnancy
Laurasen	Mrs.	610	22-Jul-1841	F	first child
Lauraton	Mrs. W. W.	944	16-Jan-1844	F	third child
Lausen	Mrs. J. H.	4934	18-Sep-1874	M	second pregnancy. "She was in a semi-unconscious & hysterical

118

Obstetrical Casebooks of Dr. F. E. Chatard – an alternative genealogical resource 1829-1883

					condition previous to birth of child & remained so for a short time after."
Law	Mrs. James	337	21-Sep-1838	F	second child
Law	Mrs. James	701	02-Apr-1842	M	fourth child
Law	Mrs. James O.	825	27-Feb-1843	M	fifth child
Law	Mrs. James O.	1184	02-Aug-1845	M	sixth child
Law	Mrs. John	366	17-Feb-1839	M	second child
Law	Mrs. John	873	02-Aug-1843	F	third child
Lawder	Mrs. Wm.	2183	26-Sep-1852	F	first child
Lawn	Mrs. Richard	2438	17-Jun-1854	M	first child
Lawn	Mrs. Richard	2772	22-Jul-1856	F	second child
Lawson	Mrs. Allen	4422	28-Feb-1869	F	first pregnancy
Lawson	Mrs. J. Herbert	5018	15-Nov-1875	F	third pregnancy
Lawson	Mrs. L. H.	4850	06-Aug-1873	F	first pregnancy
Lazaraitch [?]	Mrs. C.	3247	11-Jun-1859	M	second child
League	Mrs. G. W.	2265	09-Apr-1853	M	first child
League	Mrs. George W.	2518	30-Nov-1854	F	second child
League	Mrs. James	464	19-Feb-1840	M	11th child
Leake	Mrs.	1097	02-Jan-1845	F	first child
Leaken	Mrs. John	4430	18-Mar-1869	F	first pregnancy
Leber	Mrs. W. F.	4595	06-Oct-1870	M	first pregnancy
Leddy	Mrs. John	237	02-Jun-1837	F	third child
Ledoy	Mrs.	566	16-Jan-1841	M	
Lee	Mrs.	851	03-Jun-1843	M	colored
Lee	Mrs. A. K.	1029	29-Aug-1844	M	born 6 AM

Obstetrical Casebooks of Dr. F. E. Chatard – an alternative genealogical resource 1829-1883

Lee	Mrs. C. O'Donnell	4596	09-Oct-1870	M	first pregnancy
Lee	Mrs. C. O'Donnell	4981	01-Jun-1875		fourth pregnancy
Lee	Mrs. C. O'Donnell	5102	01-Feb-1877	M	fifth pregnancy
Lee	Mrs. C. O'Donnell	5176	20-Dec-1878	F	sixth pregnancy
Lee	Mrs. C. O'Donnell	5224	27-Sep-1880	F	seventh pregnancy
Lee	Mrs. Charles C.	3298	23-Nov-1859	F	first child
Lee	Mrs. Charles O'D.	4748	25-Apr-1872	M	second pregnancy
Lee	Mrs. Charles O'D.	4834	14-May-1873	M	third pregnancy
Lee	Mrs. Collins	786	01-Dec-1842	F	third child, stillborn
Lee	Mrs. Columbus	5181	21-Feb-1879	F	second pregnancy
Lee	Mrs. Columbus	5119	05-May-1877	M	first pregnancy
Lee	Mrs. J. Simms	1038	12-Sep-1844	M	third child
Lee	Mrs. John	670	08-Jan-1842	M	fourth child
Lee	Mrs. L. Collins	928	07-Dec-1843	F	fifth child
Leese	Mrs. Franklin	2337	21-Sep-1853	M	first child
Lefevre	Mrs. I. A.	4858	04-Oct-1873	M	fifth pregnancy
Lefevre	Mrs. J. A.	4113	07-Jul-1866	F	third pregnancy
Lehr	Mrs. Robert	4288	14-Dec-1867	F	attended by Dr. VanBibber, internal hemorrhaging,

Obstetrical Casebooks of Dr. F. E. Chatard – an alternative genealogical resource 1829-1883

child stillborn					
Leib	Mrs. J. S.	4663	16-May-1871	F	first pregnancy, miscarried 18 months ago, aged 38 years
Lelly	Mrs. J. W.	3337	07-Feb-1860	F	fourth child
Lemmon	Mrs. J. Southgate	4999	26-Aug-1875	F	second pregnancy
Lemmon	Mrs. R.	87	13-Nov-1833	F	eighth child
Lemmon	Mrs. R.	326	20-Aug-1838	M	10th child
Lenald	Mrs.	201	29-Aug-1836		attended by Dr. Bunche, second child, child dead. "The woman died two days after, I anticipated she would survive many days."
Lenmon	Mrs. Richard	602	15-Jun-1841	M	11th child
Lentz	Mrs.	879	22-Aug-1843	M	first child
Lentz	Mrs. Lewis	1851	10-Jun-1850	M	second child
Leonard	Mrs. J.	4744	15-Apr-1872	M	third pregnancy
Leonard	Mrs. Thomas	1797	20-Jan-1850	M	third child, stillborn
Leonard	Mrs. Thomas	2139	25-May-1852	F	fourth child
Leopold	Mrs. Charles	1921	29-Nov-1850	F	first child
Leopold	Mrs. Charles	2120	27-Mar-1852	M	second child
Lepper	Mrs. Charles	4347	08-Jul-1868	F	first pregnancy
Lepper	Mrs. Charles	4566	23-Jun-1870	F/F	second pregnancy, twins
Lerghan	Mrs. J.	4094	23-Mar-1866	F/F	second pregnancy
Leroy	Mrs. Philip M.	1136	10-Mar-1845	M	second child
Lerx (Letts), Jr.	Mrs. J.	2240	10-Feb-1853	F	second child
Lesene	Mrs. J. A.	3369	18-May-1860	M	first child
Lester	Mrs. Thomas	3779	25-May-1863	F	second pregnancy
Lestrange	Mrs. P.	4926	20-Aug-1874	F	second pregnancy
Lestrange	Mrs. Patrick	4781	12-Sep-1872	F	third pregnancy

Obstetrical Casebooks of Dr. F. E. Chatard – an alternative genealogical resource 1829-1883

Levenkime [?]	Mrs.	2326	28-Aug-1853	M	fourth child, attended by Dr Edward Miller
Levering	Mrs.	1015	22-Jul-1844	F	third child
Levering	Mrs. A. R.	705	10-Apr-1842	M	third child
Levering	Mrs. D.	850	19-May-1843	F	third child
Levering	Mrs. Eugene	1202	12-Sep-1845	M/	second child, twins
Levering	Mrs. Thomas	606	05-Jul-1841	F	fifth child
Levering	Mrs. Thomas	812	18-Jan-1843	F	seventh child
Levering	Mrs. Thomas	1083	04-Dec-1844	F	born about 5 PM
Lewis	Mrs. C. S.	312	10-Jul-1838	M	second child
Lewis	Mrs. C. S.	516	12-Aug-1840	F	third child, 8 pounds
Lewis	Mrs. C. S.	832	14-Mar-1843	M	fourth child
Lilly, Jr.	Mrs. Alonzo	4905	27-May-1874	M	second pregnancy
Lilly, Jr.	Mrs. Alonzo	5037	01-Feb-1876	M	third pregnancy
Lilly, Jr.	Mrs. Alonzo	5168	28-Aug-1878	M	fourth pregnancy
Liman	Mrs.	1116	05-Feb-1845	M	second child
Lind	Mrs. E. G.	3871	26-Mar-1864	M	first pregnancy
Lindsay	Mrs. W.	207	25-Sep-1836	F	eighth child, forceps delivery
Linehan	Mrs. Michael	2282	13-May-1853	F	first child
Linekamp	Mrs. J. H.	2874	06-Mar-1857	M/	premature at six months, twins, died shortly after birth
Linzey	Mrs.	70	31-Mar-1833	F	first child. "Has enjoyed uniform good health."
Lippitt	Mrs. Augustus	5091	12-Nov-1876	M	second pregnancy
Lisé	Madame	1543	22-Feb-1848	F	14th child
Littig	Mrs. John M.	5255	08-May-1882	F	first pregnancy
Littig	Mrs. Luther	2512	20-Nov-1854	M	eighth child
Littig	Mrs. P.	1102	14-Jan-1845	first child	

122

Obstetrical Casebooks of Dr. F. E. Chatard – an alternative genealogical resource 1829-1883

Lizé	Madame	1322	17-Aug-1846	M	attended by my father during my absence.
Lloyd	Mrs. B. R.	3208	13-Mar-1859	M	first child
Lloyd	Mrs. B. R.	3360	20-Apr-1860	M	second child
Lloyd	Mrs. Edward	4665	20-May-1871	M	first pregnancy
Lloyd	Mrs. Edward	4800	04-Dec-1872	F	second pregnancy
Lloyd	Mrs. W.	4796	16-Nov-1872	M	fourth pregnancy
Lloyd	Mrs. Wm.	4070	09-Jan-1866	M/F	first pregnancy, twins
Lloyd	Mrs. Wm.	4523	14-Jan-1870	M	third pregnancy
Lloyd	Mrs. Wm. J.	4309	29-Feb-1868	M	second pregnancy
Logan	Mrs. I.	4381	06-Nov-1868	F	third pregnancy, forceps delivery
Logue	Mrs.	381	28-Apr-1839	F	first child
Logue	Mrs. James	480	15-Apr-1840	M	first child
Logue	Mrs. James	837	10-Apr-1843	M	third child
Logue	Mrs. James	1088	15-Dec-1844	F	
Loney	Mrs. B. S.	2785	25-Aug-1856	M	second child
Loney	Mrs. Bodenit	2971	02-Oct-1857	F	third child, premature at eight months
Loney	Mrs. Bodinet	3158	04-Nov-1858	F	fourth child
Loney	Mrs. Bodinet	3306	15-Dec-1859	M	fifth child
Loney	Mrs. Bodinet	3492	17-Feb-1861	F	sixth child
Loney	Mrs. Thomas D.	3131	11-Sep-1858	M	third child
Loney	Mrs. W. A.	4005	13-May-1865	F	first pregnancy
Long	Mrs. J.	4419	10-Feb-1869	F	second pregnancy
Long	Mrs. J. R.	4255	15-Sep-1867	F	first pregnancy
Lopez	Mrs. J. H.	3304	12-Dec-1859	M	third child, dead
Lorghan	Mrs. John	3953	07-Dec-1864	F	first pregnancy

Obstetrical Casebooks of Dr. F. E. Chatard – an alternative genealogical resource 1829-1883

Louis	Elizabeth	362	05-Feb-1839	M	a colored woman
Love	Mrs. J. F.	4692	25-Sep-1871	F	first pregnancy
Low	Mrs.	1370	24-Dec-1846	F	second child
Lowrey	Mrs. Philip	865	09-Jul-1843	M	first child
Luckett	Mrs. James H.	2513	22-Nov-1854	F	ninth child
Lupton	Mrs.	92	23-Dec-1833	F	aged 16, first child
Lurman	Mrs.	307	25-Jun-1838	M	second child, 8.5 pounds
Lurman	Mrs. G.	1067	28-Oct-1844	M	sixth child
Lurman	Mrs. G.	1738	14-Aug-1849	M	eighth child
Lurman	Mrs. G. L.	455	08-Jan-1840	F	third child
Lurman	Mrs. G. L.	671	14-Jan-1842	F	fourth child
Lurman	Mrs. G. L.	2067	05-Dec-1851	F	ninth child
Lurman	Mrs. G. W.	2365	12-Dec-1853	F	tenth child
Lutts	Mrs. J.	2560	21-Feb-1855	F	third child
Lutts	Mrs. John	2867	23-Feb-1857	F	fourth child
Lutts	Mrs. John	3198	19-Feb-1859	F	fifth child
Lutts	Mrs. John	3506	13-Apr-1861	M	sixth child
Lutz	Mrs. N.	1928	19-Dec-1850	M	third child
Lutz	Mrs. N.	2364	09-Dec-1853	M	fourth child
Lynch	Mrs. Dennis	2730	02-Apr-1856	M/	third child, twins
Lyon	Mrs. A. J.	4403	05-Jan-1869	M	first pregnancy
Lyon	Mrs. A. J.	4579	27-Jul-1870	M	second pregnancy
Lyon	Mrs. A. J.	4941	04-Oct-1874	F	fourth pregnancy
Lyon	Mrs. J.	4056	29-Nov-1865	M	fourth pregnancy
Lyon	Mrs. James	801	31-Dec-1842	M	first child
Lyon	Mrs. P.	321	04-Aug-1838	F	first child

124

Obstetrical Casebooks of Dr. F. E. Chatard – an alternative genealogical resource 1829-1883

Lyon	Mrs. Peter	560	14-Dec-1840	F	second child
Lyon	Mrs. Saml.	4564	21-Jun-1870	F	consultation with Drs. Donaldson & Howard; mother died on 26th; child dead
Lyons	Mrs. J.	3417	11-Sep-1860	M	second child
Lyons	Mrs. J.	3760	17-Mar-1863	M	third pregnancy
Lyons	Mrs. J.	4269	24-Oct-1867	F	fifth pregnancy
Lyons	Mrs. J.	4851	04-Sep-1873	F	sixth pregnancy
Lyons	Mrs. W. B.	4493	20-Oct-1869	M	sixth or seventh pregnancy
M.	Mrs.	3357	29-Mar-1860	M	at St. Vincent's Asylum
Macdonald	Mrs. P. M.	3037	25-Jan-1858	M	second child
Macias	Mrs. Jose	4795	05-Nov-1872	M	sixth pregnancy
Macias	Mrs. J. M.	4490	05-Oct-1869	M	fifth pregnancy
Macias	Mrs. Jose	4618	05-Dec-1870	F	fifth pregnancy
Mackall	Mrs. L.	1122	13-Feb-1845	F	born 7:20 AM
Mackenzie	Mrs. G. N.	2870	03-Mar-1857	F	fourth child
Mackenzie	Mrs. Colin	2476	13-Sep-1854	M	first child
Mackenzie	Mrs. Colin	3138	01-Oct-1858	F	second child
Mackenzie	Mrs. Colin	3519	09-May-1861	M	third child
Mackenzie	Mrs. Dr. J	2790	09-Sep-1856	F	second child
Mackenzie	Mrs. G. N.	2603	20-May-1855	F	third child
Mackenzie	Mrs. John C.	3560	24-Aug-1861	F	third child
Mackenzie	Mrs. Thomas	2448	19-Jul-1854	F	fourth child
Mackenzie	Mrs. Thomas	2819	01-Nov-1856	M	fifth child
Mackenzie	Mrs. Thomas	3113	19-Aug-1858	M	sixth child
Macklin	Mrs. J. J.	2702	13-Jan-1856	F	third child
Macklin	Mrs. Jane	2119	25-Mar-1852	F	first child

125

Obstetrical Casebooks of Dr. F. E. Chatard – an alternative genealogical resource 1829-1883

Macklin	Mrs. Jane	2433	02-Jun-1854	F	second child
Macnemere	Mrs.	45	27-Mar-1832	F	second child, forceps delivery, child dead. Long record of post-partum care
Mafone [?]	Mrs. Joseph	2422	14-May-1854	M	second child. "Seven years had elapsed between her first and second child."
Magee	Mrs.	726	19-Jun-1842	F	third child
Magee	Mrs. J.	1109	26-Jan-1845	F/M	fourth child, twins
Magee	Mrs. John	459	01-Feb-1840	M	first child
Magill	Mrs. D.	1482	23-Sep-1847	F	fourth child
Magill	Mrs. Daniel	1852	10-Jun-1850	M	fifth child
Magill	Mrs. Daniel	2172	03-Sep-1852	F	sixth child
Magill	Mrs. Daniel	2567	15-Mar-1855	F	seventh child
Magill	Mrs. J. S.	1425	28-Apr-1847	F	second child
Magill	Mrs. John	1647	24-Nov-1848	F	fourth child
Magill	Mrs. John	1790	21-Dec-1849	F	fifth child
Magill	Mrs. John	2060	21-Nov-1851	M	fifth child. This child was born with one leg doubled on the abdomen, the only case of this kind I have ever seen.
Magill	Mrs. John	4955	27-Nov-1874	M	first pregnancy, attended by a midwife, forceps
Magill	Mrs. John	5019	27-Nov-1875	M	second pregnancy
Maguire	Mrs. J. T.	3993	19-Apr-1865	F	first pregnancy. "She continued well until about the 8th or 9th day when from over excitement she was attacked with puerperal mania & was removed to Mount Hope
Maguire	Mrs. Soliman	4092	15-Mar-1866	M	first pregnancy
Maguire	Mrs. Solomon	4253	08-Sep-1867	M	second pregnancy
Mahaney	Mrs. John	240	25-Jun-1837	M	second child, mother hemorrhaged but lived
Mahon	Mrs. J.	3872	28-Mar-1864	M	second pregnancy

126

Obstetrical Casebooks of Dr. F. E. Chatard – an alternative genealogical resource 1829-1883

Mahoney	Mrs. John	147	24-May-1835	M	first child, "The child was feeble & with difficulty revived."
Maiden [?]	Mrs. Jesse	2279	12-May-1853	M	seventh child
Makin	Mrs.	581	05-Apr-1841	M	still born
Malloy	Mrs. L.	4632	07-Jan-1871	M	second pregnancy, "the child lived but a few days."
Malloy	Mrs. Laurence	4420	18-Feb-1869	F	first pregnancy
Malloy	Mrs. Laurence	4802	09-Dec-1872	M	third pregnancy, child was stillborn
Maloney	Mrs. I.	4753	13-May-1872	F	first pregnancy
Maloy	Mrs. Mary	3787	21-Jun-1863	M	at St. Vincent's Insane Asylum, first pregnancy. Child died in a few days
Mancks	Mrs. Andrew	4672	01-Jul-1871	F	ninth pregnancy
Mann	Mrs. Charles	2683	26-Nov-1855	M	fifth child
Mann	Mrs. Wm.	1906	29-Oct-1850	F	second child
Manning	Mrs. J.	4147	03-Oct-1866		sixth pregnancy, attended by Dr. Yates and Dr. Andre, child dead
Manning	Mrs. James	2515	24-Nov-1854	M	first child
Manning	Mrs. James	2887	06-Apr-1857	M	second child
Manning	Mrs. W. S.	3166	20-Nov-1858	F	first child, forceps deliver, mother died in one hour
Manquet	Mary	1098	03-Jan-1845	F	third child
Maquette	Mary	1950	25-Feb-1851	M	premature 5 months
March	Mrs. Washington	262	03-Oct-1837		early labor 28 Sept, rest & cold lemonade; aborted
March	Mrs. Washington	383	09-May-1839	M	first child
March	Mrs. Washington	917	04-Nov-1843	F	third child
March	Mrs. Washington	1132	21-Feb-1845	F	fourth child

127

Obstetrical Casebooks of Dr. F. E. Chatard – an alternative genealogical resource 1829-1883

Marchand	Mrs. Capt. J.	3674	26-Aug-1862	F	fourth child
Marchand	Mrs. Capt. J. B.	3244	01-Jun-1859	M	second child
Marchand	Mrs. Margaret	2984	20-Oct-1857	F	first child
Marchand	Mrs. Margaret	3431	20-Oct-1860	M	third child
Marden	Mrs. Jesse	609	21-Jul-1841	F	fifth child
Marden	Mrs. Jesse	858	18-Jun-1843	F	sixth child
Marden	Mrs. Jesse	1296	25-Jun-1846	F	sixth child
Marelius	Mrs.	2009	05-Aug-1851	M	first child
Marge	Mrs. G. T.	936	25-Dec-1843	F	second child
Markin	Mrs.	1152	16-May-1845	F	fourth child
Marnen	Mrs. J.	3390	01-Jul-1860	M	first child
Marriott	Mrs.	3452	02-Dec-1860	M	first child
Marriott	Mrs. Geo.	89	24-Nov-1833	M	seventh child, 7.5 pounds
Marriott	Mrs. J. McKim	1917	20-Nov-1850	F	second child
Marriott	Mrs. John McKim	2338	27-Sep-1853	M	third child
Marriott	Mrs. W. McKim	2760	15-Jun-1856	M	fourth child
Marsh	Mrs. Ch. H.	3897	17-Jun-1864	M	first pregnancy
Marshall	Mrs.	62	08-Jan-1833	M	third child, seven pounds
Marshall	Mrs.	3469	24-Dec-1860	M	at St. Vincent's Asylum, fifth child
Marshall	Mrs. D. Baxtor	5067	14-Jul-1876	F	first pregnancy, forceps delivery
Marshall	Mrs. Luke	2915	12-Jun-1857	F	fourth child
Marsters	Mrs. J. D.	1631	13-Oct-1848	F	third child
Martens	Mrs. J. D.	2987	25-Oct-1857	F	seventh child
Martin	Henrietta	159	05-Oct-1835	F	colored woman, fifth child

128

Obstetrical Casebooks of Dr. F. E. Chatard – an alternative genealogical resource 1829-1883

Martin	Mrs.	397	16-Jul-1839			colored.
Martin	Mrs. Charles	1932	04-Jan-1851		M	first child
Martin	Mrs. Charles	2164	04-Aug-1852		F	second child
Martin	Mrs. Charles	2346	20-Oct-1853		F	third child
Martin	Mrs. Charles	3028	30-Dec-1857		F	fourth child
Martin	Mrs. George	313	12-Jul-1838		F	fourth child
Martin	Mrs. Henrietta	269	08-Nov-1837		F	a colored woman
Martin	Mrs. J.	897	30-Sep-1843		M	third child
Martin	Mrs. Major	1641	06-Nov-1848		F	third child
Martin	Mrs. Major	1966	03-Apr-1851		F	fourth child
Martin	Mrs. Major	2277	07-May-1853		M	fourth child
Martin	Mrs. Paul	1228	14-Nov-1845		F	first child
Martin	Mrs. Paul	1403	15-Mar-1847		F	second child
Martin	Mrs. Paul	1873	05-Aug-1850			third child. Labor induced by an attack of no mark of the disease
Martine	Mrs. Jacob	1607	01-Aug-1848		M	first child
Mason	Mrs.	248	29-Aug-1837		F	fifth child
Mason	Mrs.	522	15-Sep-1840		M	first child
Mason	Mrs. Charles	4399	29-Dec-1868		F	first pregnancy, "The child died the next day & very suddenly."
Mason	Mrs. Charles	4603	28-Oct-1870		M	second pregnancy
Mason	Mrs. D.	4062	20-Dec-1865		F	fourth pregnancy
Mason	Mrs. Joseph	3180	08-Jan-1859		M	sixth child
Mason	Mrs. P.	251	03-Sep-1837		M	second child, spina bifida & hydrocephalus
Mason	Mrs. Peter	501	17-Jun-1840		M	fifth child, has club foot
Mason	Mrs. Peter	629	27-Aug-1841		M	sixth child, 4-6 months, died
Mason	Mrs. Peter	800	24-Dec-1842		M	premature labor, child died

Obstetrical Casebooks of Dr. F. E. Chatard – an alternative genealogical resource 1829-1883

Mason	Mrs. Wm.	981	02-Apr-1844	F	third child
Mason	Mrs. Wm.	1303	07-Jul-1846	F	fourth child
Mason	Mrs. Wm.	1475	09-Sep-1847	M	first child
Mason	Mrs. Wm.	1565	21-Apr-1848	F	fifth child
Mason	Mrs. Wm.	1869	04-Aug-1850	M	sixth child
Massicott	Mrs. Robert	2889	10-Apr-1857	F	third child
Massicott	Mrs. Robert	3616	10-Feb-1862	M	first child
Mastenon	Mrs.	16	17-Jul-1830		first child
Masters	Mrs. J. D.	1458	31-Jul-1847	M	second child
Masters	Mrs. J. D.	2601	25-May-1855	M	sixth child
Mathews	Mrs. Stockdale	2686	30-Nov-1855	F	first child
Mathews	Mrs. Wm.	1935	11-Jan-1851	F	first child
Matthews	Mrs. Mary	1622	28-Sep-1848	M	first child
Mauck	Mrs. John	2092	27-Jan-1852	F	second child
Mauglin, Jr.	Mrs. W. W.	4983	07-Jun-1875	M	second pregnancy
Maulsby	Mrs. Wm. P.	1784	09-Dec-1849	M	eighth child
Maurer	Mrs. R. S>	3689	15-Oct-1862	F	second child
Maxwell	Mrs. Alexander	2616	08-Jul-1855	F	third child. "The child was almost asphyxiated."
Maxwell	Mrs. John	2167	23-Aug-1852	F	first child
May	Miss	3775	28-Apr-1863	M	at St. Vincent's Asylum, first pregnancy
May	Mrs.	29	13-Oct-1831		first child, mother very sick with convulsions; attended by elder Dr. Chatard. "The child was extracted extremely weak & brought to only by friction with brandy"
May	Mrs.	73	01-May-1833	M	see 13 Oct 1831 [#29], second child, eight months, 6.75 lbs
May	Mrs.	140	29-Mar-1835		see 1 May 1833 [#73], abortion of seven weeks, hemorrhage

Obstetrical Casebooks of Dr. F. E. Chatard – an alternative genealogical resource 1829-1883

May	Mrs.	180	13-Feb-1836	M	see 1 May 1833 [#73], third child. Mother died 4:30 PM 22 Feb. Long description of care
May	Mrs. Domenic	2993	10-Nov-1857	F	second child
May	Mrs. Domenick	2712	12-Feb-1856	M	first child
May	Mrs. Domenick	4007	20-May-1865	M	fourth pregnancy
May	Mrs. E.	666	27-Dec-1841	M	third child
May	Mrs. Edward	474	27-Mar-1840	F	second child
May	Mrs. Edward	898	02-Oct-1843	M	fourth child
May	Mrs. Ferdinand	4373	01-Oct-1868	F	first pregnancy
May	Mrs. M.	331	28-Aug-1838	F	first child, eight months, still born
May	Mrs. Phillip	4590	26-Sep-1870	M	first pregnancy
May	Mrs. Phillip	4720	11-Dec-1871	M	second pregnancy
Mayer	Mrs. Brantz	1215	14-Oct-1845	F	fifth child. She was attacked on the fourth day with puerperal fever and died the 17th day after her confinement
Mayer	Mrs. Henry	822	19-Feb-1843	F	first child
Maynard	Mrs. Warren	3900	03-Jul-1864	M	first pregnancy
Maynard	Mrs. Warren	4058	03-Dec-1865	M	second pregnancy
McAleer	Mrs.	1788	16-Dec-1849	M	third child
McAleer	Mrs. John	2021	27-Aug-1851	F	fourth child
McAleer	Mrs. John	2254	15-Mar-1853	F	fifth child
McAleer	Mrs. Phillip H.	5096	08-Jan-1877	M	first pregnancy
McAleese	Mrs.	318	25-Jul-1838	F	born at 5 PM
McAleese	Mrs.	760	14-Sep-1842	M	born 1 AM
McAleese	Mrs.	1131	20-Feb-1845	M	born 5:20 AM
McAleese	Mrs. A.	1452	10-Jul-1847	M	ninth child
McAroy	Mrs. Hugh	588	21-Apr-1841	F	ninth child

131

Obstetrical Casebooks of Dr. F. E. Chatard – an alternative genealogical resource 1829-1883

McArthey	Mrs. Timothy	2664	03-Oct-1855	F	second child
McAvey [?]	Mrs. H.	354	06-Dec-1838	M	eighth child
McAvey [?]	Mrs. Paul	2693	23-Dec-1855	F	first child
McAvoy	Mrs.	205	18-Sep-1836	F	seventh child
McAvoy	Mrs. Dennis	3191	23-Jan-1859	M/	second child, twins
McAvoy	Mrs. Dennis	3934	08-Oct-1864	F	third pregnancy
McAvoy	Mrs. Dennis	4342	15-Jun-1868	F	fifth pregnancy. "The child was alive when born but did not survive many minutes."
McAvoy	Mrs. Dennis	4601	23-Oct-1870	F	fifth pregnancy
McAvoy	Mrs. P.	3117	25-Aug-1858	F	third child
McAvoy	Mrs. Paul	2894	24-Apr-1857	M	second child
McAvoy	Mrs. Paul	3613	05-Feb-1862	M	fifth child
McAvoy	Mrs. Paul	3933	08-Oct-1864	F	fifth pregnancy
McAvoy	Mrs. Paul	4551	25-May-1870		sixth pregnancy
McCabe	Mrs.	1165	10-Jun-1845	M	first child, stillborn
McCabe	Mrs.	1342	11-Oct-1846	F	third child, forceps delivery, stillborn
McCabe	Mrs. John	4896	13-Apr-1874	F	ninth pregnancy
McCadon	Mrs.	22	23-Apr-1831		second child
McCafferty	Catherine	228	22-Mar-1837	M	second child
McCafferty	Mrs. A.	1301	29-Jun-1846	M	seventh child
McCafferty	Mrs. A.	1623	01-Oct-1848	M	first child
McCafferty	Mrs. Elizabeth	1355	14-Nov-1846	F	second child
McCaffray	Catherine	356	26-Dec-1838	F	third child
McCaffray	Mrs. Catherine	558	10-Dec-1840	F	fourth child
McCaffray	Mrs. George	4124	27-Jul-1866	F	first pregnancy

132

McCaffray	Mrs. George	5243	20-Nov-1881	F	"a tedious labour, called to assist my son. We decided to apply the forceps"
McCaffray	Mrs. Henry	2134	21-May-1852	F	second child
McCaffray	Mrs. Henry	2456	02-Aug-1854	F	third child
McCaffray	Mrs. Henry	2808	16-Oct-1856	F	fourth child
McCaffray	Mrs. Henry	3122	28-Aug-1858	M	fifth child
McCaffray	Mrs. Henry	3608	22-Jan-1862	F	sixth child
McCaffray	Mrs. Henry	3876	04-Apr-1864	M	seventh pregnancy
McCaffray	Mrs. Henry	4480	17-Aug-1869	F	eighth pregnancy
McCaffrey	Mrs. Henry	1864	26-Jul-1850	F/F	first child, twins, second child died
McCann	Mrs.	138	06-Mar-1835		"Found the child partly delivered, the legs protruding …", six months, child dead
McCann	Mrs.	1114	30-Jan-1845	M	first child
McCann	Mrs.	1288	02-Jun-1846		second child
McCann	Mrs.	1381	20-Jan-1847	F	first child
McCann	Mrs.	1582	31-May-1848	M	second child
McCann	Mrs.	1808	02-Feb-1850	F	third child
McCann	Mrs. C.	2300	03-Jul-1853	M	fifth child
McCann	Mrs. Charles	2061	22-Nov-1851	M	fourth child
McCann	Mrs. Charles	2613	05-Jul-1855	F	sixth child
McCann	Mrs. Charles	3049	26-Feb-1858	F	seventh child
McCAnn	Mrs. John	5133	27-Jun-1877	F	first pregnancy
McCann	Mrs. R.	2015	16-Aug-1851	F	second child
McCann	Mrs. Richard	1619	23-Sep-1848	F	first child
McCarthy	Mrs. J.	4525	25-Jan-1870	F	second pregnancy

Obstetrical Casebooks of Dr. F. E. Chatard – an alternative genealogical resource 1829-1883

McCarthy	Mrs. Thomas	4514	16-Dec-1869	M	ninth pregnancy
McCarthy	Mrs. Timothy	4799	29-Nov-1872	F	tenth pregnancy
McCartney	Mrs. Patrick	1556	25-Mar-1848	M	first child
McClanahan	Mrs.	142	04-Apr-1835		an abortion about ten weeks
McClellan	Mrs. W.	1392	08-Feb-1847	M	fifth child
McClelland	Mrs. George	4659	08-May-1871	F	fourth pregnancy, consultation with Dr. W. Griffith
McClelland	Mrs. George	5164	29-Jul-1878	M	fifth pregnancy
McClelland	Mrs. J. S.	4838	15-Jun-1873	F	second pregnancy
McClennan	Mrs. Rose	814	24-Jan-1843	M	third child
McCloskey	Mrs. Wm.	1558	05-Apr-1848	F	fourth child
McColgan	Mrs. Dennis	2197	26-Oct-1852	F	first child
McColgan	Mrs. Dennis	2532	28-Dec-1854	F	second child
McComas	Mrs.	618	04-Aug-1841	F	born about 1 PM
McComas	Mrs. J.	3960	18-Dec-1864	F	first pregnancy
McComas	Mrs. J.	4142	03-Sep-1866		second pregnancy
McComas	Mrs. J.	4321	04-Apr-1868	F	third pregnancy " … the cord produced the death of the child."
McComas	Mrs. Kesiah	1306	14-Jul-1846	F	third child
McConnell	Mrs. Patrick	3378	30-May-1860	M	third child
McCormick	Mrs. Alexander	2339	27-Sep-1853	M	second child
McCormick	Mrs. J.	4050	13-Nov-1865	M	first pregnancy
McCormick	Mrs. J.	4568	25-Jun-1870	F	third pregnancy
McCormick	Mrs. J. H.	4055	27-Nov-1865	M	third pregnancy, forceps delivery
McCormick	Mrs. James	3048	21-Feb-1858	M	third child
McCormick	Mrs. John	4285	01-Dec-1867	M	second pregnancy
McCormick	Mrs. John	4832	09-May-1873	F	fourth pregnancy

Obstetrical Casebooks of Dr. F. E. Chatard – an alternative genealogical resource 1829-1883

McCormick	Mrs. John	5123	24-May-1877	M	fifth pregnancy
McCormick	Mrs. John H.	3756	08-Mar-1863	F	first pregnancy
McCormick	Mrs. Margaret	2099	08-Feb-1852	M	first child
McCoy	Mrs. Harry	4217	04-May-1867	M	second pregnancy
McCoy	Mrs. Harry	4400	30-Dec-1868		third pregnancy. "The child was delivered by forceps on account of the feeble condition of the mother."
McCoy	Mrs. Harry	4573	15-Jul-1870	F	fourth pregnancy. Mother died 6:30 AM from hemorrhage
McCoy	Mrs. R. H.	4311	06-Mar-1868	F	third pregnancy
McCrandon	Mrs.	532	14-Oct-1840		delivered with forceps
McCronie	Mrs. Michael	4080	13-Feb-1866	F	fourth pregnancy
McCubbin	Mrs.	428	29-Oct-1839	M	third child
McCubbin	Mrs. William	3516	04-May-1861	F	first child
McCubbin	Mrs. WM.	3875	03-Apr-1864	F	second pregnancy
McCullogh	Mrs. John	4100	09-May-1866	M	second pregnancy
McCulloh	Mrs. J. S.	1181	28-Jul-1845	M	first child
McCulloh	Mrs. J. S.	1544	24-Feb-1848	F	second child
McCullough	Mrs. John	3704	12-Nov-1862	M	first child, forceps delivery
McCurley	Mrs. J.	965	05-Mar-1844	F	first child
McDermott	Mrs. Wm.	790	09-Dec-1842	M	tenth child
McDonald	Mrs. A.	468	18-Mar-1840	F	first child
McDonald	Mrs. A. A.	597	28-May-1841	F	second child
McDonald	Mrs. A. A.	933	11-Dec-1843	M	premature birth
McDonald	Mrs. A. A.	1079	24-Nov-1844	F	fourth child
McDonald	Mrs. James	2908	03-Jun-1857	M	fourth child
McDonald	Mrs. James	3984	08-Feb-1865	M	seventh pregnancy

Obstetrical Casebooks of Dr. F. E. Chatard – an alternative genealogical resource 1829-1883

McDonald	Mrs. Mary	1603	22-Jul-1848	F	first child
McDonald	Mrs. Michael	5057	12-Jun-1876	M	first pregnancy
McDonald	Mrs. Patrick	1810	07-Feb-1850	F	second child
McDonald	Mrs. Patrick	2106	01-Mar-1852	M	third child
McDowell	Mrs. E. G.	4681	22-Jul-1871	F	fifth pregnancy, child was dead
McDowell	Mrs. R.	1189	07-Aug-1845	F	fourth child
McElderry	Mrs. Henry	1065	26-Oct-1844	M	eighth child
McElroy	Mrs. G. W.	1290	08-Jun-1846	F	second child
McElroy	Mrs. George	2298	20-Jun-1853	M	fifth child
McElroy	Mrs. George	2645	30-Aug-1855	M	sixth child
McElroy	Mrs. George	3054	09-Mar-1858	M	seventh child
McElroy	Mrs. George W.	1579	19-May-1848	F	third child
McElroy	Mrs. George W.	1848	01-Jun-1850	F	fourth child
McElroy	Mrs. P.	1207	25-Sep-1845	M	seventh child
McElroy	Mrs. P.	1367	18-Dec-1846	M	third child
McFaden	Mrs. Patrick	1593	30-Jun-1848	M	sixth child
McFaden	Mrs. Patrick	1938	24-Jan-1851	F	seventh child
McFaul	Mrs.	348	06-Nov-1838	F	
McFaul	Mrs. Eneas	997	30-May-1844	M	fifth child
McFaul	Mrs. James	661	30-Nov-1841	F	first child
McFaul, Jr.	Mrs. Eneas	533	15-Oct-1840	M	
McFaul, Jr.	Mrs. Eneas	696	22-Mar-1842	F	born 5 AM
McFaul, Sr.	Mrs. Eneas	382	29-Apr-1839	M	10th child
McFaul, Sr.	Mrs. Eneas	485	02-May-1840	M	11th child
McFaul, Sr.	Mrs. Eneas	764	29-Sep-1842	M	born about 5 AM

Obstetrical Casebooks of Dr. F. E. Chatard – an alternative genealogical resource 1829-1883

McGahan	Mrs. John	1428	01-May-1847	M	fifth child
McGann	Mrs.	752	27-Aug-1842	M	fourth child
McGee	Mrs.	203	12-Sep-1836	M	second child
McGee	Mrs.	271	07-Dec-1837	M	first child
McGee	Mrs. Francis	1862	07-Jul-1850	F	sixth child, stillborn, attended by Dr. Porter
McGee	Mrs. J.	3947	24-Nov-1864	F/F	first pregnancy, twins, stillborn
McGill	Mrs.	753	28-Aug-1842	M	second child
McGill	Mrs. D.	1175	07-Jul-1845	M	third child
McGill	Mrs. G.	907	21-Oct-1843	M	fourth child
McGill	Mrs. J.	1757	29-Sep-1849	M	"mother of many children."
McGinn	Mrs. James	2210	24-Nov-1852	M	sixth child
McGinn	Mrs. James	2764	28-Jun-1856		attended by Dr Buckleman. Died fourth day
McGinnerty	Mrs.	42	22-Jan-1832	F	see 7 Jan 1830. Third child
McGinnerty	Mrs.	90	26-Nov-1833	F	see 22 Jan 1832 [#42], fourth child
McGinnis	Mrs.	1507	05-Dec-1847	M	second child
McGinnity	Mrs.	7	07-Jan-1830	M	aged 22, second child
McGiven	Mrs. J.	1799	22-Jan-1850	M	born 9 AM
McGlanchlie	Mrs. Dennis	4098	08-Apr-1866	M	first pregnancy
McGlauchlin	Mrs. Dennis	4272	29-Oct-1867	F	second pregnancy
McGlauchlin	Mrs. James	3568	10-Sep-1861	M	first child, forceps delivery
McGlellan	Mrs. J.	2218	11-Dec-1852	F	second child
McGlennan	Mrs.	1644	15-Nov-1848	M	first child
McGlennan	Mrs. A.	4922	16-Aug-1874	M	second pregnancy
McGlennan	Mrs. Alexis	4772	24-Jul-1872	M	first pregnancy
McGlennan	Mrs. Alexius	5059	19-Jun-1876	M	third pregnancy

Obstetrical Casebooks of Dr. F. E. Chatard – an alternative genealogical resource 1829-1883

McGloan	Mrs.	647	28-Oct-1841	M	fourth child
McGlone	Mrs. Thomas	3214	20-Mar-1859	F	first child
McGowan	Mrs. Henry	2435	08-Jun-1854	M	second child
McGowan	Mrs. Henry	3050	01-Mar-1858	M	fourth child
McGowan	Mrs. Henry	3421	27-Sep-1860	M	fifth child
McGowan	Mrs. Henry	3885	27-Apr-1864	M	sixth pregnancy
McGowan	Mrs. Henry	4091	14-Mar-1866	F	seventh pregnancy
McGowan	Mrs. Mary	2149	18-Jun-1852	F	first child
McGreevy	Mrs. H.	4946	01-Nov-1874	F	fourth pregnancy
McGreevy	Mrs. Hamilton	4779	10-Sep-1872	M	third pregnancy
McGuire	Mrs. Thomas	2066	04-Dec-1851	M	fifth child
McGurk	Mrs. Margaret	1604	24-Jul-1848	M	first child, stillborn
McHenry	Mrs. James	111	18-Jul-1834	M	"She has suffered during this pregnancy from swelling in inferior extremities."
McHenry	Mrs. W. R.	2407	21-Mar-1854	F	third child
McHenry	Mrs. W. R.	2703	20-Jan-1856	F	fourth child
McHenry	Mrs. Wm. R.	2073	14-Dec-1851	F	second child
McIlvaine	Mrs. W. J.	4483	24-Aug-1869	M	second pregnancy
McIntire	Jane	11	10-Mar-1830	F	third child
McKanna	Mrs.	1203	12-Sep-1845	F	first child
McKee	Mrs.	1335	21-Sep-1846	F	first child
McKee	Mrs. Francis	4106	27-May-1866	M	third pregnancy
McKee	Mrs. John	1702	21-Apr-1849	F	second child
McKee	Mrs. John	2224	25-Dec-1852	M	third child
McKee	Mrs. M. F.	3259	26-Jul-1859	M	first child
McKee	Mrs. M. F.	3551	06-Aug-1861	F	second child

138

Obstetrical Casebooks of Dr. F. E. Chatard – an alternative genealogical resource 1829-1883

McKeever	Mrs. J.	315	20-Jul-1838	F	third child
McKeever	Mrs. James	3914	31-Jul-1864	M	first pregnancy
McKeever	Mrs. John	475	31-Mar-1840	M	
McKeever	Mrs. John	1035	02-Sep-1844	M	child was born when I arrived
McKeever	Mrs. Joseph	3892	28-May-1864	M	second pregnancy
McKeever	Mrs. Joseph E.	3695	28-Oct-1862	M	first child
McKenna	Margaret	3450	28-Nov-1860	F	at St. Vincent's Asylum, first child
McKenna	Mrs. P. J.	4965	29-Dec-1874	M	second pregnancy, "It made but little progress & the patient plead for relief, I applied the forceps."
McKenna	Mrs. Thomas		04-Mar-1872	F	fourth pregnancy
McKenna	Mrs. Thomas	4135	13-Aug-1866	M	first pregnancy
McKenna	Mrs. Thomas	4358	04-Aug-1868	M	second pregnancy
McKenna	Mrs. Thomas	4499	05-Nov-1869	F	third pregnancy
McKenna	Mrs. Thomas	4825	28-Mar-1873	F/F	fifth pregnancy, twins
McKenna	Mrs. Thomas	4900	03-May-1874	F	sixth pregnancy
McKenna	Mrs. Thomas	5027	02-Jan-1876	F	seventh pregnancy
McKenna	Mrs. Thomas	5124	03-Jun-1877	F	eighth pregnancy
McKenna	Mrs. Thomas	5163	19-Jul-1878	F	ninth pregnancy
McKenna	Mrs. Thomas	5249	25-Mar-1882	M	12th pregnancy
McKenne	Mrs. Edward	2574	30-Mar-1855	F	third child, dead
McKenny	Mrs.	38	29-Dec-1831	M	first child
McKenny	Mrs.	164	10-Nov-1835	F	first child
McKenzie	Mrs. Dr. John	2347	20-Oct-1853	M	first child
McKiever	Mrs. John	709	16-Apr-1842	M	born 8:30 PM
McKim	Mrs. Haslett	795	18-Dec-1842	M	first child

139

Obstetrical Casebooks of Dr. F. E. Chatard – an alternative genealogical resource 1829-1883

McKim	Mrs. Isaac	3380	10-Jun-1860	M	first child, forceps delivery. "She complained of not being able to see a short time before applying the forceps & that state continued after the conclusion of labour …"
McKim	Mrs. Isaac	3585	09-Nov-1861	F	second child
McKim	Mrs. Isaac	3940	02-Nov-1864	M	third pregnancy
McKin	Mrs. J. S.	707	15-Apr-1842	M	fourth child
McKinley	Mrs. William	2525	13-Dec-1854	M	first child
McKinley	Mrs. William	3266	01-Sep-1859	F	fourth child
McKinley	Mrs. Wm.	2853	15-Jan-1857	F	second child
McKinley	Mrs. Wm.	3584	08-Nov-1861	M	fourth child
McKinley	Mrs. Wm.	4061	14-Dec-1865	F	fifth pregnancy
McKitterick	Mrs. P.	1566	23-Apr-1848	F	13th child
McLane	Mrs. W. H.	1286	29-May-1846	M	born a little before 6 PM
McLane	Mrs. W. H.	1416	03-Apr-1847	F/M	sixth child, twins
McLane	Mrs. Wm. H.	1115	02-Feb-1845	F	born 6 PM
McLean	Mrs.	565	14-Jan-1841	M	second child
McLean	Mrs. W.	2543	20-Jan-1855	M	fourth child
McLear	Mrs.	333	12-Sep-1838	F	first child
McMahon	Mrs. J.	3313	28-Dec-1859	M	second child
McMahon	Mrs. John	2786	29-Aug-1856	F	first child
McMahon	Mrs. John	3640	20-May-1862	F	third child
McMahon	Mrs. P.	4616	04-Dec-1870	M	first pregnancy
McMahon	Mrs. P.	4812	24-Jan-1873	F	third pregnancy
McMahon	Mrs. P.	4891	21-Mar-1874	M	fourth pregnancy
McMahon	Mrs. Patrick	4721	22-Dec-1871	F	second pregnancy
McMahon	Mrs. Patrick	5213	22-Jan-1880	M/F	fifth pregnancy, twins

Obstetrical Casebooks of Dr. F. E. Chatard – an alternative genealogical resource 1829-1883

McMahon	Mrs. S.	3171	09-Dec-1858	F	fourth child. "The child gave no signs of life."
McMahon	Mrs. S. M.	3849	30-Jan-1864	M	fifth pregnancy
McManus	Mrs. Patrick	3382	14-Jun-1860	M	third child
McMullan	Mrs. John	4737	03-Mar-1872	F	first pregnancy
McMullen	Mrs. J.	4844	01-Jul-1873	F	second pregnancy
McMullen	Mrs. J.	5055	14-May-1876	F	fourth pregnancy
McMullen	Mrs. J. F.	5184	16-May-1879	M	fifth pregnancy
McMullen	Mrs. John	4954	26-Nov-1874	M	third pregnancy
McMurray	Mrs. Samuel	192	07-Jul-1836	F	child born after an hour
McNally	Mrs. Henry	3851	26-Jan-1864	M	first pregnancy
McNally	Mrs. Henry	4929	02-Sep-1874	F	first pregnancy, forceps delivery
McNally	Mrs. Henry R.	5041	19-Feb-1876	M	second pregnancy
McNally	Mrs. James	563	05-Jan-1841	M	third child
McNally	Mrs. James	892	19-Sep-1843	F	first child
McNally	Mrs. James	1160	29-May-1845	M	second child
McNally	Mrs. James	1418	06-Apr-1847	M	third child
McNally	Mrs. James	1725	13-Jul-1849	F	sixth child
McNally	Mrs. James	2597	18-May-1855	M	sixth child
McNally	Mrs. James	2977	09-Oct-1857	M	seventh child
McNally	Mrs. James	3620	12-Mar-1862	F	eighth child
McNally	Mrs. James F.	5008	04-Oct-1875	M	second pregnancy
McNally	Mrs. John	3854	06-Feb-1864	M	sixth pregnancy, attended by Dr. Dalrymple
McNally	Mrs. John	4161	29-Nov-1866	F/F	first pregnancy
McNally	Mrs. John	4305	09-Feb-1868	F	second pregnancy
McNally	Mrs. P.	3487	07-Feb-1861	F	second child, child dead
McNally	Mrs. Thomas	1793	08-Jan-1850	F/F	attended by Dr. Perkins. Twins, one stillborn

Obstetrical Casebooks of Dr. F. E. Chatard – an alternative genealogical resource 1829-1883

McNamara	Mrs.	4256	15-Sep-1867	F	fifth pregnancy
McNamee	Mrs. J. F.	4606	03-Nov-1870	M	first pregnancy
McNaughton	Mrs. Mary	441	25-Nov-1839		retained placenta for 57 hours
McNeal	Mrs. Joshua V.	5142	07-Aug-1877	F	forceps delivery
McNeal	Mrs. Michael	4835	15-May-1873	M	first pregnancy
McNeil	Mrs.	639	06-Oct-1841	F	first child
McNeill	Mrs. T.	4244	25-Aug-1867	M	first pregnancy
McNier	Mrs. Michael	3143	06-Oct-1858	F	first child
McPharmin	Mrs. Margaret	2213	30-Nov-1852	M	first child
McShane	Mrs. J.	4735	03-Feb-1872	F	second pregnancy
McShane	Mrs. John	4584	07-Sep-1870	F	first pregnancy
McShane	Mrs. John	4852	05-Sep-1873	F	third pregnancy
McShane	Mrs. John	5081	26-Sep-1876	F	fifth pregnancy
McShea	Mrs. Charles	2995	10-Nov-1857	F	first child. " … the pains were very violent."
McTavish	Mrs. Alexander	2983	19-Oct-1857	M	first child
McTavish	Mrs. Carroll	2672	25-Oct-1855	F	second child
McTavish	Mrs. Carroll	2885	31-Mar-1857	M	third child
McTavish	Mrs. Carroll	3192	25-Jan-1859	F	fourth child
Meakins	Mrs. J.	4194	19-Feb-1867	F	fourth pregnancy
Medcalfe	Mrs. Edward	481	17-Apr-1840	M	second child
Medcalfe	Mrs. Edward	1826	27-Feb-1850	F	fourth child
Medtart	Mrs. J.	293	27-Mar-1838	F	first child
Medtart	Mrs. Jesse	463	16-Feb-1840	F	second child
Meer	Mrs.	2125	21-Apr-1852	F	second child
Meer	Mrs. John	2374	06-Jan-1854	F	third child

142

Obstetrical Casebooks of Dr. F. E. Chatard – an alternative genealogical resource 1829-1883

Meer	Mrs. John	2757	08-Jun-1856	M	fourth child
Meer	Mrs. John	3148	19-Oct-1858	M	fifth child
Meer	Mrs. John	3534	16-Jun-1861	M	sixth child
Meer	Mrs. John	3827	05-Dec-1863	M	seventh pregnancy
Meer	Mrs. Michael	4362	07-Aug-1868	F	first pregnancy
Memmert	Mrs.	2122	14-Apr-1852	M	first child, seven months premature
Memmert	Mrs.	2248	23-Feb-1853	M	second child
Merceret	Mrs. Francis	2649	05-Sep-1855	F	first child
Merceret	Mrs. Lewis	2520	02-Dec-1854	M	third child. "The child lived about two months."
Merceret	Mrs. Louis	1973	06-May-1851	F	first child
Merceret	Mrs. Louis	2235	28-Jan-1853	M	second child
Merceret	Mrs. Louis	2813	23-Oct-1856	M	fourth child
Merceret	Mrs. Louis	3080	02-May-1858	F	fourth child
Merceret	Mrs. Louis	3294	17-Nov-1859	F	sixth child
Merceret	Mrs. Louis	3708	20-Nov-1862	M	seventh child
Merceret	Mrs. Louis	3833	29-Dec-1863	F	eighth pregnancy
Meredith	Mrs.	1787	15-Dec-1849	M	second child
Meredith	Mrs. Morris	2924	23-Jun-1857	M	third child
Mering	Mrs. Edward	3066	06-Apr-1858	M	first child
Merry	Mrs. Jasper M.	2674	26-Oct-1855	M	second child
Merryman	Mrs.	860	23-Jun-1843	F	first child
Merryman	Mrs. Oliver P.	1199	31-Aug-1845	F	second child
Merryman	Mrs. Oliver P.	1493	20-Oct-1847	M	third child
Merryman	Mrs. R. S.	4610	19-Nov-1870	M	first pregnancy
Merryman	Mrs. Richard S.	4782	17-Sep-1872	M	second pregnancy
Meyer	Mrs. A. Karl	5153	26-Mar-1878	F	first pregnancy, forceps delivery

143

Obstetrical Casebooks of Dr. F. E. Chatard – an alternative genealogical resource 1829-1883

Meyer	Mrs. A. Karl	5203	08-Oct-1879	F	second pregnancy, forceps delivery
Miale	Mrs. Henry	4586	14-Sep-1870	M	fourth pregnancy
Michael	Mrs.	423	09-Oct-1839	M	first child
Michael	Mrs.	782	25-Nov-1842	M	second child
Micthell	Mrs. J.	571	27-Jan-1841	F	first child
Middleton	Mrs. Wm.	4714	04-Dec-1871	M	first pregnancy
Miles	Mrs.	617	02-Aug-1841	M	ninth child
Miles	Mrs. Hugh	956	06-Feb-1844	M	born five o'clock PM
Miles	Mrs. S.	841	24-Apr-1843	M	tenth child, 9 1/2 pounds
Miles	Mrs. Uriah	556	08-Dec-1840	F	fourth child
Miles	Mrs. Uriah	750	24-Aug-1842	M	fifth child
Miles	Mrs. Wm.	1444	11-Jun-1847	F	12th child
Miller	Mrs.	3888	16-May-1864	F	first pregnancy
Miller	Mrs. J.	4827	01-Apr-1873	M	third pregnancy
Miller	Mrs. Jacob	4937	23-Sep-1874	F	fourth pregnancy
Miller	Mrs. Joshua	4444	30-Apr-1869	M	first pregnancy
Miller	Mrs. Joshua	4619	10-Dec-1870	M	second pregnancy
Miller	Mrs. W. H.	3395	16-Jul-1860	M	third child
Miller	Mrs. W. H.	3946	21-Nov-1864	M	fifth pregnancy
Miller	Mrs. William	2976	09-Oct-1857	M	second child
Miller	Mrs. Wm.	250	01-Sep-1837	M	born 4 PM
Miller, Jr.	Mrs. Wm.	2685	29-Nov-1855	M	first child
Milligan	Mrs. G. B.	2647	03-Sep-1855	M	second child
Milligan	Mrs. G. B.	3111	06-Aug-1858	F	third child
Milligan	Mrs. G. B.	3406	12-Aug-1860	F	fourth child
Milligan	Mrs. George	3683	23-Sep-1862	M	fourth child

Obstetrical Casebooks of Dr. F. E. Chatard – an alternative genealogical resource 1829-1883

Milligan	Mrs. George	3982	04-Feb-1865	F	fifth pregnancy
Milligan	Mrs. Sophia	2403	18-Mar-1854	F	first child
Millington	Mrs.	56	23-Oct-1832	F	third child, eight pounds
Mills	Mrs. James	1058	18-Oct-1844	M/F	first child, twins
Milner	Mrs. J. K.	4188	10-Feb-1867	F	sixth pregnancy
Milner	Mrs. J. P.	3319	09-Jan-1860	F	Nr. 271 Pratt Street, first child
Milner	Mrs. J. P.	3858	24-Feb-1864	M	fifth pregnancy
Milner	Mrs. John	2363	08-Dec-1853	M	first child
Milner, Jr.	Mrs. J. P.	3118	26-Aug-1858	M	second child
Milnor	Mrs. J. K.	2963	13-Sep-1857	M	third child
Mintell	Mrs. Elizabeth	2371	28-Dec-1853	M	first child
Mintell	Mrs. James	3263	21-Aug-1859	M	second child
Miskelly	Mrs. Sylvester	1998	11-Jul-1851	M	third child
Miskelly	Mrs. Sylvester	2273	28-Apr-1853	F	fourth child
Missionier	Madame Felix	3884	27-Apr-1864	M	fifth pregnancy
Mitchell	Mrs.	114	09-Aug-1834		fifth child, breech
Mitchell	Mrs.	195	28-Jul-1836	M	first child
Mitchell	Mrs. A.	2261	01-Apr-1853	M	first child
Mitchell	Mrs. Francis J.	3035	16-Jan-1858	M	fourth child
Mitchell	Mrs. Joseph	737	18-Jul-1842	M	second child, difficult birth, mother died 4 PM
Mitchell	Mrs. R. J.	3218	27-Mar-1859	F	second child
Mitchell	Mrs. Robert J.	2969	23-Sep-1857	F	first child
Mittan	Mrs. J. P.	974	25-Mar-1844	M	fifth child
Moale	Mrs. Edward	3924	14-Sep-1864	F	first pregnancy
Moale	Mrs. Henry	3793	20-Jul-1863	F	first pregnancy

145

Obstetrical Casebooks of Dr. F. E. Chatard – an alternative genealogical resource 1829-1883

Moale	Mrs. Henry	4051	17-Nov-1865	M	second pregnancy
Moale	Mrs. Henry	4284	30-Nov-1867	F	third pregnancy
Moale	Mrs. Henry	5104	05-Feb-1877	M	sixth pregnancy
Moguet [see	Mrs. Nelson	856	17-Jun-1843	F	colored, second child
Molly	Mrs. Wm.	3785	17-Jun-1863	M	third pregnancy
Monaghan	Mrs. John	1262	17-Feb-1846	F	second child
Monahan	Mrs. John	3802	14-Aug-1863	F	third pregnancy
Monquet	Mary	630	28-Aug-1841	M	colored, first child
Monquet	Mary	1689	16-Mar-1849	M	fifth child
Montell	Mrs. James	3581	04-Nov-1861	F	third child, forceps delivery
Montell	Mrs. James	3837	05-Jan-1864	M/	fourth pregnancy, twins
Montell	Mrs. James	4019	20-Aug-1865	M	fifth pregnancy
Montell	Mrs. James E.	980	31-Mar-1844	M	first child, mother died on 9 April 1844
Montgomery	Mrs.	1659	04-Jan-1849	F	fourth child
Moore	Mrs. James H.	2246	22-Feb-1853	M	first child
Moore	Mrs. William	2826	17-Nov-1856	F	first child
Moquett	Mary	1408	25-Mar-1847	F	fourth child
Morgan	Mrs.	116	08-Sep-1834	M	first child
Morgan	Mrs.	1391	05-Feb-1847	M	third child
Morgan	Mrs. Charles	2288	04-Jun-1853	M	fourth child
Morly	Mrs. J.	3340	09-Feb-1860	M	first child
Morris	Mrs. John	1805	29-Jan-1850	F	third child
Morris	Mrs. John B.	5033	21-Jan-1876	F	fourth pregnancy, 7.5 months. "Her previous pregnancy continued full ten months."
Morris	Mrs. John E.	4146	01-Oct-1866	M	first pregnancy, attended by Dr. Patterson
Morris, Jr.	Mrs. John B.	4847	21-Jul-1873	M	third pregnancy, previous gestation was 10 months

Obstetrical Casebooks of Dr. F. E. Chatard – an alternative genealogical resource 1829-1883

Morrison	Mrs. J. L.	4263	09-Oct-1867	M	first pregnancy, attended by Dr. Hartman, child hydrocephalic. "Mother remained unconscious & died on 9th."
Morse	Mrs. T.	3742	26-Jan-1863	M	fifth child
Morse	Mrs. Thomas S.	3020	18-Dec-1857	M	first child
Mortimer	Mrs. J. W.	3133	24-Sep-1858	M	third child
Mortimer	Mrs. John W.	3311	26-Dec-1859	M	fourth child
Morton	Mrs. George	592	01-May-1841	M	sixth child
Morton	Mrs. George	437	13-Nov-1839	F	fifth child
Morton	Mrs. George	818	13-Feb-1843	F	seventh child
Morton	Mrs. George	1101	12-Jan-1845	F	ninth child
Morton	Mrs. George	1499	21-Nov-1847	F	ninth child
Morton	Mrs. George	1912	11-Nov-1850	F	tenth child
Morton	Mrs. George C.	2177	10-Sep-1852	M	11th child
Morton	Mrs. Samuel P.	4405	11-Jan-1869	M	fifth pregnancy
Motley	Mrs. W.	3414	07-Sep-1860	M	first child
Motley	Mrs. William	4723	23-Dec-1871	M	eighth pregnancy
Motley	Mrs. Wm.	3606	21-Jan-1862	F	second child
Motley	Mrs. Wm.	4119	17-Jul-1866	M	fifth pregnancy
Motley	Mrs. Wm.	4479	15-Aug-1869	M	seventh pregnancy
Mowenckel	Mrs. H. P.	3046	21-Feb-1858	F	sixth child
Mowenckle	Mrs. H. P.	3277	28-Sep-1859	F	eighth child
Moylen	Mrs. James	3334	27-Jan-1860	F	first child
Moylon	Mrs. Michael	3623	02-Apr-1862	M	eighth child
Mudge	Mrs. A. B.	1040	13-Sep-1844	M	second child
Mudge	Mrs. A. B.	1266	15-Mar-1846	F	third child
Mudge	Mrs. A. B.	1515	20-Dec-1847	F	fourth child

147

Surname	Given	ID	Date	Sex	Notes
Mudge	Mrs. A. B.	1765	18-Oct-1849	M	fifth child
Mudge	Mrs. A. B.	2024	06-Sep-1851	F	sixth child
Mudge	Mrs. A. B.	2264	07-Apr-1853	M	seventh child
Mudge	Mrs. A. B.	2475	07-Sep-1854	F	eighth child
Mudge	Mrs. A. B.	3152	23-Oct-1858	M	eighth child
Mudge	Mrs. A. B.	3347	04-Mar-1860	M	11th child
Mudge	Mrs. Harry	4761	12-Jun-1872	F	first pregnancy
Mudge	Mrs. Harry	4909	17-Jun-1874	F	second pregnancy
Mudge	Mrs. Harry	5011	16-Oct-1875	M	third pregnancy
Mullan	Mrs. Bernard	3836	04-Jan-1864	F	seventh pregnancy
Mullen	Mrs. Bernard	3290	05-Nov-1859	M	sixth child. "The infant died on the eighth day apparently of heart affection."
Mullen	Mrs. J.	3339	08-Feb-1860	M	second child
Mullen	Mrs. Timothy	3780	05-Jun-1863	F	first pregnancy
Muller	Mrs. B.	2170	30-Aug-1852	M/	twins, first stillborn
Muller	Mrs. B.	2417	29-Apr-1854	F	second child
Muller	Mrs. Barney	2689	14-Dec-1855	M	third child
Muller	Mrs. Barney	2947	12-Aug-1857	M	fifth child
Muller	Mrs. J.	3464	13-Dec-1860	F	third child
Muller	Mrs. J.	3996	25-Apr-1865	M	first pregnancy, "labor was very difficult … the child was dead."
Muller	Mrs. John	2401	08-Mar-1854	F	second child
Muller	Mrs. Michael A.	4685	03-Aug-1871	F	first pregnancy
Muller	Mrs. Thomas	1696	29-Mar-1849	M	first child
Mullin	Mrs. J.	3596	03-Dec-1861	F	fourth child
Mullin	Mrs. J.	4036	29-Sep-1865	M	fifth pregnancy
Mullin	Mrs. John	3226	03-May-1859	M	first child

148

Obstetrical Casebooks of Dr. F. E. Chatard – an alternative genealogical resource 1829-1883

Mullin	Mrs. Michael	4780	11-Sep-1872	M	second pregnancy
Mullin	Mrs. Michael A.	4892	23-Mar-1874	F	third pregnancy
Muncaster	Mrs.	391	12-Jun-1839	M	second child
Muncaster	Mrs.	901	12-Oct-1843	M	third child
Munck	Mrs. Andrew	2871	04-Mar-1857	M	third child
Munck	Mrs. Andrew	3741	25-Jan-1863	M/F	fourth child, twins
Munck	Mrs. Andrew	3956	10-Dec-1864	F	seventh pregnancy
Munck	Mrs. Andrew	4377	12-Oct-1868	F	eighth pregnancy
Munck	Mrs. John	2383	19-Jan-1854	M	third child
Munck	Mrs. John	3425	07-Oct-1860	M	sixth child
Munck	Mrs. John	4160	25-Nov-1866	M	seventh pregnancy
Munck	Mrs. L. A.	2450	24-Jul-1854	M	second child
Muncks	Mrs. Andrew	1760	08-Oct-1849	M	first child
Muncks	Mrs. John	2840	12-Dec-1856	M	fourth child
Muncks	Mrs. John	3220	28-Mar-1859	F	fifth child
Munek	Mrs. John	1885	08-Sep-1850	M	first child
Murdoch	Mrs. A.	690	03-Mar-1842	F	eighth child
Murdoch	Mrs. Alexander	448	01-Jan-1840	F	seventh child
Murdoch	Mrs. Campbell	4546	11-May-1870	M	second pregnancy
Murdoch	Mrs. Dr. Russell	5135	02-Jul-1877	F	third pregnancy
Murdoch	Mrs. W. F.	364	12-Feb-1839	M	12th child
Murdoch	Mrs. W. F.	494	28-May-1840	F	13th child
Murdoch	Mrs. W. F.	708	15-Apr-1842	F	14th child
Murdoch	Mrs. A.	131	30-Dec-1834		abortion two months, hemorrhage
Murdock	Mrs. A.	272	21-Dec-1837	F	fifth child

149

Obstetrical Casebooks of Dr. F. E. Chatard – an alternative genealogical resource 1829-1883

Murdock	Mrs. Campbell	4374	02-Oct-1868	F	first pregnancy
Murdock	Mrs. W. F.	294	02-Apr-1838	F	eleventh child
Murphy	Mrs.	2	08-Sep-1829	M	19 years old, first child, attended by midwife Mrs. Faithful; bled her about 25 oz; "delivered of a stout boy weighing 7 2/4 lb."
Murphy	Mrs. Dennis	4029	10-Sep-1865	F	first pregnancy
Murphy	Mrs. Pierce	2146	09-Jun-1852	M	first child
Murray	Mrs.	434	09-Nov-1839	M	first child
Murray	Mrs.	1920	28-Nov-1850	M	attended by Dr. O'Donnell, difficult birth, forceps
Murray	Mrs. Abraham	819	14-Feb-1843	F	born 2:30 AM
Murray	Mrs. Frank	5103	03-Feb-1877	M	first pregnancy
Murray	Mrs. Frank	5185	19-Mar-1879	M	second pregnancy, attended by a midwife
Murray	Mrs. J. C.	817	04-Feb-1843	F	fourth child
Murray	Mrs. James	567	19-Jan-1841	F	second child
Murray	Mrs. James	797	19-Dec-1842	M	fifth child
Murray	Mrs. John	584	06-Apr-1841	M	second child
Murray	Mrs. John	2752	21-May-1856	M	first child
Murray	Mrs. Michael	5195	12-Jul-1879	M	first pregnancy
Murray	Mrs. Michael	5237	22-Jun-1881	F	second pregnancy
Murray	Mrs. Patrick	611	24-Jul-1841	M	first child
Murray	Mrs. Patrick	809	17-Jan-1843	M	second child
Murray	Mrs. R. C.	438	15-Nov-1839	M	third child
Murray	Mrs. Thomas		14-Jul-1859	F	third child
Murray	Mrs. Thomas	67	17-Feb-1833	F	third child, eight months, child dead; Long description of care
Murray	Mrs. Thomas	96	09-Feb-1834	F	see 17 Feb 1833 [#67], fourth child, spina bifida, feet deformed, child died 19 Apr 1834

Obstetrical Casebooks of Dr. F. E. Chatard – an alternative genealogical resource 1829-1883

Murray	Mrs. Thomas	268	07-Nov-1837	F	born 6:30 PM
Murray	Mrs. Thomas	2465	17-Aug-1854	F	first child
Murray	Mrs. Thomas	2822	13-Nov-1856	M	second child
Murray	Mrs. Thomas	3688	10-Oct-1862	M	fourth child
Muth	Mrs. M. J.	5265	23-Apr-1883	M	14th pregnancy
Myers	Jane	1942	05-Feb-1851	M	colored. Second child
Myers	Mrs. A.	2189	09-Oct-1852	M	first child
Myers	Mrs. A. J.	4510	05-Dec-1869	M	third pregnancy
Myers	Mrs. August	4488	26-Sep-1869	M	second pregnancy
Myers	Mrs. Augustus	4303	03-Feb-1868	M	first pregnancy
Myers	Mrs. Humphrey	2372	29-Dec-1853	M	second child
Myers	Mrs. Humphrey	2751	21-May-1856	F	third child
Myers	Mrs. Humphrey	3141	04-Oct-1858	M	fourth child
Myers	Mrs. J. P.	4260	26-Sep-1867	F	first pregnancy
Myers	Mrs. James	4294	08-Jan-1868	F	second pregnancy
Myers	Mrs. John	2268	16-Apr-1853	F	first child, died at birth
Myers	Mrs. W. H.	2315	04-Aug-1853	M	third child
Mylen	Mrs. James	2625	29-Jul-1855	F	fourth child
Nash	Mrs. Catherine	497	10-Jun-1840	M	born 10:30 PM
Neal	Mrs. A.	637	23-Sep-1841	M	third child
Neal	Mrs. Abner	943	15-Jan-1844	M	fourth child
Neal	Mrs. R.	418	10-Sep-1839	F	second child
Neale	Mrs. Clarence	4443	30-Apr-1869	F	second pregnancy
Neale	Mrs. Harry	4505	24-Nov-1869	M	second pregnancy. "…virulent pain in the extreme lower border of the right iliac region … was relieved by a hypodermic injection of morphine."

151

Obstetrical Casebooks of Dr. F. E. Chatard – an alternative genealogical resource 1829-1883

Neeland	Mrs.	133	27-Jan-1835	M	second child
Neff	Mrs.	144	29-Apr-1835	F	second child
Neidlip	Mrs. Augustine	3670	15-Aug-1862	M	second child
Neigarth	Mrs. F.	926	01-Dec-1843	M	fourth child
Neilson	Mrs. Albert	4545	11-May-1870	F	second pregnancy
Neilson	Mrs. George	1110	26-Jan-1845	M	premature, four months
Neilson	Mrs. R.	694	16-Mar-1842	M	second child
Neimeyer	Mrs. J. H.	1341	26-Sep-1846	F	first child
Neimyer	Mrs. H.	2762	19-Jun-1856	F	seventh child
Neimyer	Mrs. J. H.		01-Jun-1858		four month pregnant
Neimyer	Mrs. J. H.	1505	30-Nov-1847	F	second child
Neimyer	Mrs. J. H.	1999	12-Jul-1851	M	fourth child
Neimyer	Mrs. J. H.	2242	18-Feb-1853	M	fifth child
Neimyer	Mrs. J. H.	2443	03-Jul-1854	M	sixth child
Nequenez [?]	Mrs.	323	14-Aug-1838	M	attended by Justin Power
Neugent	Mrs. William	2251	02-Mar-1853	M	first child
Nevin	Mrs. John	4410	24-Jan-1869	M	second pregnancy
Newport	Mrs. R. M.	3905	14-Jul-1864	M	first pregnancy, attended by Dr. John Buckler, forceps delivery
Nicholson	Mrs C. G.	3772	20-Apr-1863	F	first pregnancy
Nicholson	Mrs. J. H. R.	4580	28-Jul-1870	F	first pregnancy
Nicholson	Mrs. J.H.R.	4739	08-Mar-1872	M	second pregnancy
Nicholson	Mrs. Thomas	2863	18-Feb-1857	F	"… the child was born when I arrived."
Nicholson	Mrs. Thomas	3176	20-Dec-1858	M	seventh child
Nicholson	Mrs. Thomas	3526	18-May-1861	F	eighth child
Nickesser	Mrs. T.	2811	20-Oct-1856	F	first child

Obstetrical Casebooks of Dr. F. E. Chatard – an alternative genealogical resource 1829-1883

Nicols	Mrs. C.	346	04-Nov-1838	M	second child, weight 12 pounds
Nidlip [Nidliss]	Mrs. A.	3878	10-Apr-1864	M	third pregnancy
Nielson	Mrs. T.	594	02-May-184_	F	first child, 7 months
Niernsee	Mrs.	1706	09-May-1849	M	fourth child
Niernsee	Mrs.	1761	09-Oct-1849	F	born 5:15 AM
Niernsee	Mrs. J. R.	2187	06-Oct-1852	M	fifth child
Niernsee	Mrs. J. R.	2588	26-Apr-1855	F	sixth child
Niersie	Mrs.	1243	29-Dec-1845	F	third child
Nigles	Mrs. Augustine	3376	28-May-1860	F	first child
Nimmo	Mrs.	2888	07-Apr-1857	M	born 1:15 PM
Nipper	Mrs. Capt. J. E.	1993	24-Jun-1851	M	seventh child
Nixon	Mrs. John	4172	29-Dec-1866	F	first pregnancy
Nixon	Mrs. John	4733	14-Jan-1872	M	fourth pregnancy
Nolan	Mrs.	1964	21-Mar-1851	F	first child, stillborn
Nones	Mrs.	2110	08-Mar-1852	F	fourth child
Nonges	Mrs. Joseph	358	06-Jan-1839	F	fourth child
Nongess	Mrs. Joseph	253	07-Sep-1837	M	third child
Nongues	Mrs.	72	19-Apr-1833	M	first child
Nongues	Mrs.	166	21-Nov-1835	F	see 19 Apr 1833 [#72], second child
Nongues	Mrs. Joseph	754	31-Aug-1842	M	sixth child
Nongues	Mrs. Joseph	1233	04-Dec-1845	F	born about 7:30 AM
Norkmans	Mrs. Juliette	2176	09-Sep-1852	F	first child
Norman	Mrs. M. S.	1311	02-Aug-1846	F	third child
Norman	Mrs. S.	4114	07-Jul-1866	F	third pregnancy
Norris	Mrs. John S.	919	11-Nov-1843	M	third child
Norris	Mrs. Sam	572	31-Jan-1841	M	first child, attended by Dr Handy & Dr Baxley

153

Obstetrical Casebooks of Dr. F. E. Chatard – an alternative genealogical resource 1829-1883

Norris	Mrs. Sidney	1162	02-Jun-1845	F	third child
Norris	Mrs. Sidney	1402	13-Mar-1847		fourth child
Norwood	Mrs. Lambert	1099	04-Jan-1845	M	first child
Nottingham	Mrs. Alonzo	5190	12-May-1879	M	first pregnancy
Nouval [?]	Mrs. Gustave	4931	10-Sep-1874	M	second pregnancy
Nowlin	Mrs. F.	83	08-Sep-1833	M	third child
Nugent	Mrs. J.	3859	25-Feb-1864	F	seventh pregnancy
Nugent	Mrs. J.	4008	26-May-1865	F	eighth pregnancy
Nugent	Mrs. J.	4460	20-Jun-1869	F	tenth pregnancy
Nugent	Mrs. J.	4676	10-Jul-1871	F	11th pregnancy
Nugent	Mrs. John	4804	14-Dec-1872	F	12th pregnancy, child dead, mother died on fourth child
Nunn	Mrs. Stephen	4139	29-Aug-1866	M	second pregnancy
Nunn	Mrs. Stephen	4398	29-Dec-1868	F	third pregnancy
Nunn	Mrs. Stephen	4643	09-Feb-1871	F	fourth pregnancy
Nunn	Mrs. Stephen	4854	15-Sep-1873	M	fifth pregnancy
Nunn	Mrs. Stephen	5179	28-Jan-1879	F	seventh pregnancy
Nunn	Mrs. Stephen	5242	07-Sep-1881	M	eighth pregnancy
Nunn	Mrs. Stephen E.	5073	04-Aug-1876	F	sixth pregnancy
Oakford	Mrs. John D.	5085	17-Oct-1876	M	first pregnancy, forceps delivery
Obendorf	Mrs. Julius	3974	15-Jan-1865	F	first pregnancy
O'Brien	Mrs. J.	1434	18-May-1847	F	seventh child
O'Brien	Mrs. John	1676	16-Feb-1849	F	eighth child
O'Brien	Mrs. John	2058	14-Nov-1851	F	ninth child
O'Brien	Mrs. Patrick	2241	13-Feb-1853	M	ninth child
O'Brien	Mrs. Thomas	2179	12-Sep-1852	F	second child

154

Obstetrical Casebooks of Dr. F. E. Chatard – an alternative genealogical resource 1829-1883

O'Brien	Mrs. Thomas	2409	27-Mar-1854	M	third child
O'Connell	Mrs.	740	29-Jul-1842	F	born about 4 AM
O'Connell	Mrs. Patrick	3658	15-Jul-1862	M	fourth child
O'Connell	Mrs. Patrick	3826	28-Nov-1863	M	fifth pregnancy
O'Connor	Mrs. John	2470	27-Aug-1854	F	second child
O'Connor	Mrs. Maria	2897	10-May-1857	M	seventh child
O'Donnell	Mrs.	247	28-Aug-1837	F	first child, stillborn
O'Donnell	Mrs. C. Oliver	4332	15-May-1868	M	first pregnancy, forceps delivery
O'Donnell	Mrs. C. Oliver	4476	08-Aug-1869	F	second pregnancy, forceps delivery
O'Donnell	Mrs. C. Oliver	4599	18-Oct-1870	M/	third pregnancy, seven months, triplets all dead
O'Donnell	Mrs. Columbus	3154	30-Oct-1858	M	first child
O'Donnell	Mrs. John	568	22-Jan-1841	M	second child, hemorrhaged
O'Donnell	Mrs. Oliver	4705	19-Nov-1871	F	fourth pregnancy, "… at her request I applied the forceps."
O'Donnell, Jr	Mrs. Columbus	3333	26-Jan-1860	M	second child
O'Donnell, Jr.	Mrs. Columbus	3525	17-May-1861	F	third child
O'Donohal	Mrs. J. H.	3552	07-Aug-1861	M	second child
Oelrichs	Mrs. Henry	1850	08-Jun-1850	M	third child
Oelrichs	Mrs. Henry	2488	27-Sep-1854	F	sixth child
Oelrichs	Mrs. Henry	2838	08-Dec-1856	M	sixth child
Oelrichs	Mrs. Henry	3121	27-Aug-1858	M	seventh child
Oelricks	Mrs. Henry	2173	04-Sep-1852	F	fourth child
O'Farrell	Mrs.	1758	29-Sep-1849	M	second child
Ogden	Mrs. J. W.	2718	02-Mar-1856	M	first child
O'Keefe	Mrs. J.	4079	08-Feb-1866	F	fifth pregnancy
Oliver	[--?--]	221	15-Jan-1837		colored woman

155

Obstetrical Casebooks of Dr. F. E. Chatard – an alternative genealogical resource 1829-1883

Surname	Given	#		Date	Sex	Notes
Oliver	Mary	8				colored, third child
Oliver	Mary	54	F	29-Sep-1832	M	see 1830 [#8]; colored, fourth child. "The child was dead and all efforts to resuscitate him were in vain."
Oliver	Mary	102		11-Apr-1834	M	see 29 Sep 1832 [#54], fifth child
Oliver	Mrs.	1776		21-Nov-1849	M	fourth child
Oliver	Mrs. John	2117		23-Mar-1852	M	12th child, stillborn
Oliver	Mrs. John	2507		08-Nov-1854	F	13th child
Oliver	Mrs. Thomas	380		26-Apr-1839	F	
O'Loughlin	Mrs. S. W.	4432		23-Mar-1869	F	fourth pregnancy
O'Loughlin	Mrs. Samuel W.	3816		17-Oct-1863	M	first pregnancy. "It had an extensive hair lip."
O'Loughlin	Mrs. William	4273		30-Oct-1867	F	third pregnancy
O'Mara	Mrs.	1747		13-Sep-1849	F	second child
O'Neil	Mrs. Jane	2320		14-Aug-1853	F	first child
O'Neil	Mrs. John	3727		31-Dec-1862	F	seventh child
O'Neill	Mrs. J.	2418		05-May-1854	M	second child
O'Neill	Mrs. J. F.	4097		05-Apr-1866	F	third pregnancy
O'Neill	Mrs. J. F.	4297		25-Jan-1868	F	fourth pregnancy
O'Neill	Mrs. J. F>	4539		23-Apr-1870	F	fifth pregnancy
O'Neill	Mrs. John F.	3274		16-Sep-1859	M	eighth child
O'Neill	Mrs. M.	3341		18-Feb-1860	M	third child
O'Neill	Mrs. Michael	3024		22-Dec-1857	F	second child
O'Neill	Mrs. Michael	3565		03-Sep-1861	M	fourth child
O'Neill	Mrs. Owen	3041		07-Feb-1858	F	first child
Orndorff	Mrs.	388		03-Jun-1839	F	first child
Orndorff	Mrs.	582		05-Apr-1841	F	second child, hemorrhage

Obstetrical Casebooks of Dr. F. E. Chatard – an alternative genealogical resource 1829-1883

Ortwein	Mrs.	914	31-Oct-1843	F	first child
Osborn	Mrs.	665	12-Dec-1841	M	fourth child
Ould	Mrs. L.	1022	13-Aug-1844	F	first child
Ould	Mrs. Lancaster	1734	29-Jul-1849	F	second child
Ould	Mrs. Lancaster	1909	05-Nov-1850	M	third child
Ould	Mrs. Lancaster	2206	17-Nov-1852	M	fourth child
Owens	Mrs. Joseph A.	1407	25-Mar-1847	F	third child
Owings	Mrs. Charles	2617	09-Jul-1855	M	second child
Page	Mrs. William	3159	05-Nov-1858	F	second child
Page	Mrs. William	3514	30-Apr-1861	M	second child
Pagels	Mrs. Edward	4943	08-Oct-1874	F	third pregnancy
Pagels	Mrs. G. H.	1240	14-Dec-1845	F	third child
Pagels	Mrs. G. H.	1460	04-Aug-1847	M	fourth child
Pagels	Mrs. G. H.	1898	08-Oct-1850	F/F	sixth child, twins
Pagles	Mrs.	747	18-Aug-1842	M	first child
Pagles	Mrs.	913	30-Oct-1843	F	second child
Pagles	Mrs. Edward	4509	04-Dec-1869	F	second pregnancy
Pagles	Mrs. G. H.	1692	20-Mar-1849	F	fourth child
Paini	Mrs. Joseph	3419	19-Sep-1860	M	second child
Palmer	Mrs. Dr. J.	1807	31-Jan-1850	F	fifth child
Palmer	Mrs. Dr. J.	2828	20-Nov-1856	F	sixth child
Palmer	Mrs. J. W.	4725	25-Dec-1871	M	second pregnancy, "An interval of fourteen years having elapsed between her two pregnancies."
Palmer	Mrs. Thomas	2794	21-Sep-1856	F	first child
Palmer	Mrs. W.	975	26-Mar-1844	M	rapid labor, seven months

157

Obstetrical Casebooks of Dr. F. E. Chatard – an alternative genealogical resource 1829-1883

Pancoast	Mrs.	983	09-Apr-1844		first child
Parks	Mrs. Sophia	530	12-Oct-1840		called to assist Dr. Roberts, mother recovered
Parr, Jr.	Mrs. Preston	4515	19-Dec-1869	F	second pregnancy, premature at 8 months
Parrish	Mrs.	4020	20-Aug-1865	M	second pregnancy, attended by Dr. Kepler, prolonged labor
Parrott	Mrs. E.	521	23-Aug-1840	M	
Parrott	Mrs. W. J.	689	01-Mar-1842	M	born 7 PM
Partridge	Mrs. James	1611	09-Aug-1848	F	first child
Partridge	Mrs. James L.	2020	25-Aug-1851	F	third child
Passano	Mrs. J. F.	4640	30-Jan-1871	F	first pregnancy
Passano	Mrs. J. F.	4859	04-Oct-1873	M	second pregnancy
Passano	Mrs. Joseph F.	5038	01-Feb-1876	M	third pregnancy
Patella	Mrs. Felix	4963	19-Dec-1874	F	second pregnancy
Patridge	Mrs. J.	1786	13-Dec-1849	F	second child
Patterson	Mrs. Henry	748	23-Aug-1842	M	first child
Patterson	Mrs. Henry	1006	25-Jun-1844	M	second child
Patterson	Mrs. Henry	1567	23-Apr-1848	M/F	fourth child, twins
Patterson	Mrs. Henry	1843	18-May-1850	M	fourth child
Patterson	Mrs. Henry	2214	05-May-1852	F	sixth child
Patterson	Mrs. Henry	2691	18-Dec-1855	F	fifth child, attended by Dr Rielly
Patterson	Mrs. W.	502	19-Jun-1840	M	difficult birth
Patterson	Mrs. W.	5219	22-May-1880	M	second pregnancy, forceps delivery
Patterson	Mrs. William	5042	03-Mar-1876	F	first pregnancy, slow labour, forceps hyxiated
Patterson	Mrs. William	5251	07-Apr-1882	F	third pregnancy, forceps delivery
Pattison	Mrs. Thomas	4011	02-Jun-1865	F	seventh pregnancy
Pattison	Mrs. Thomas	4245	25-Aug-1867	F	eighth pregnancy

158

Obstetrical Casebooks of Dr. F. E. Chatard – an alternative genealogical resource 1829-1883

Patton	Mrs.	607	07-Jul-1841	F	first child, stillborn
Paul	Mrs. D'Arcy	3353	17-Mar-1860	M	first child
Payne	Mrs. George H.	5089	07-Nov-1876	M	first pregnancy
Payne	Mrs. J.	3761	20-Mar-1863	F	11th pregnancy
Payne	Mrs. J. J.	2055	11-Nov-1851	M	born 10 AM
Payne	Mrs. J. J.	2439	19-Jun-1854	F	seventh child
Payne	Mrs. J. J.	2806	09-Oct-1856	M	born 7:30 PM
Payne	Mrs. J. J.	3183	15-Jan-1859	F	ninth child
Payne	Mrs. J. J.	3485	01-Feb-1861	F	tenth child
Payne	Mrs. J. J.	4293	01-Jan-1868	M	12th pregnancy
Paynter	Mrs. N. W.	2608	25-Jun-1855	M	second child
Paynter	Mrs. N. W.	3240	24-May-1859	M	third child
Paynter	Mrs. W.	3429	15-Oct-1860	M	fourth child
Pearce	Mrs. Nathaniel	32	30-Oct-1831	F	Camden Street. Third child; six pounds
Pearson	Mrs.	1170	25-Jun-1845	M	first child
Pearson	Mrs. Andrew	682	07-Feb-1842	M	fifth child
Pearson	Mrs. T. R.	1838	25-Apr-1850	M	second child
Peletar	Mrs. William	81	15-Aug-1833	F	third child
Pendleton	Mrs.	763	24-Sep-1842	F	born 3:30 AM
Pendleton	Mrs. W. N.	1086	08-Dec-1844	F	eighth child
Penniman	Mrs. A.	811	18-Jan-1843	F	second child
Penniman	Mrs. R.	1981	31-May-1851	M	second child
Penniman	Mrs. W. R.	2262	05-Apr-1853	M	third child
Penniman	Mrs. Wm.	2592	11-May-1855	F	fourth child
Penniman	Mrs. Wm. R.	1796	17-Jan-1850	F	first child
Penniman	Mrs. Wm. R.	3388	24-Jun-1860	M	fifth child

159

Obstetrical Casebooks of Dr. F. E. Chatard – an alternative genealogical resource 1829-1883

Penniman	Mrs. Wm. R.	3723	28-Dec-1862	M	sixth child
Pennington, Jr.	Mrs Josiah	4090	11-Mar-1866	M	seventh pregnancy
Perine	Mrs. Wm. B.	3680	19-Sep-1862	F	first child
Perkins	Mrs. James	2777	05-Aug-1856	M	second child
Perkins	Mrs. James	3059	18-Mar-1858	F	third child
Perkins	Mrs. James	3289	02-Nov-1859	F	fourth child
Perkins	Mrs. James	4145	30-Sep-1866	M	seventh pregnancy
Perkins	Mrs. Otis	1255	01-Feb-1846		forceps birth, stillborn. Mother died following day
Perkins	Mrs. Wm. H.	3477	16-Jan-1861	F	first child
Perkins	Mrs. Wm. H.	3668	11-Aug-1862	M	second child
Perram	Mrs.	222	30-Jan-1837	F	second child
Perry	Mrs.	34	20-Nov-1831	F	residence at Pierce Alley, fourth child
Perry	Mrs.	148	02-Jun-1835	M	see 20 Nov 1831 [#34], sixth child
Perry	Mrs. Roger	3082	14-May-1858	F	first child
Petri	Mrs.	694	20-Mar-1842	F	fourth child
Petri	Mrs.	887	07-Sep-1843	F	fifth child
Petri	Mrs.	1443	10-Jun-1847	M	difficult birth
Petry	Mrs.	319	31-Jul-1838	M	second child
Petry	Mrs. R.	465	24-Feb-1840	M	third child
Pfifer	Mrs. P.	733	04-Jul-1842	F	first child, attended by Dr. Collins
Phelps	Mrs. A.	769	22-Oct-1842	F	second child
Phelps	Mrs. E.	583	06-Apr-1841	F	first child
Phelps	Mrs. E.	1070	05-Nov-1844	M	third child
Phelps	Mrs. J.	4693	29-Sep-1871	F	second pregnancy
Phelps	Mrs. James G.	4441	23-Apr-1869	F	first pregnancy

Obstetrical Casebooks of Dr. F. E. Chatard – an alternative genealogical resource 1829-1883

Phenix	Mrs. Howard	2425	19-May-1854	F	first child
Phenix	Mrs. Howard	2722	09-Mar-1856	M	second child
Phillips	Mrs Edward	3335	31-Jan-1860	F	fifth child
Phillips	Mrs.	985	23-Apr-1844	F	second child, forceps delivery
Phillips	Mrs.	1875	08-Aug-1850	F	fifth child
Phillips	Mrs. Edward	2113	15-Mar-1852	F	first child
Phillips	Mrs. Edward	2429	29-May-1854	F	second child, stillborn, difficult birth
Phillips	Mrs. Edward	2951	22-Aug-1857	F	fourth child
Phillips	Mrs. Edward	3504	07-Apr-1861	M	sixth child
Phillips	Mrs. Edward	3694	27-Oct-1862	M	sixth child
Phillips	Mrs. Edward	3868	18-Mar-1864	F	eighth pregnancy
Phillips	Mrs. Edward	4562	18-Jun-1870	M	ninth pregnancy
Phillips	Mrs. Edward C.	2652	07-Sep-1855	M	third child
Phillips	Mrs. J. E.	3167	26-Nov-1858	F	first child
Phillips	Mrs. J. E.	3348	05-Mar-1860	F	Nr. 8 Parkin St., second child
Phillips	Mrs. James	2768	13-Jul-1856	M	first child
Phillips	Mrs. John	2697	31-Dec-1855	F	first child, dead
Phillips	Mrs. John	2895	05-May-1857	M	second child
Phillips	Mrs. John	3351	12-Mar-1860	M	third child
Phillips	Mrs. John	3819	13-Nov-1863	M	fourth pregnancy
Phillips	Mrs. John E.	4044	30-Oct-1865	F	third pregnancy
Phillips	Mrs. Thomas	1679	23-Feb-1849	M	second child, stillborn
Phillips	Mrs. Thomas	1982	01-Jun-1851	M	third child
Phillips	Mrs. Thomas	2835	01-Dec-1856	M	fifth child
Phillips	Mrs. J. B.	4673	03-Jul-1871	F	fourth pregnancy
Philpot	Mrs.	301	09-May-1838	F	first child after 9 years marriage

Obstetrical Casebooks of Dr. F. E. Chatard – an alternative genealogical resource 1829-1883

Piccioli	Mrs.	885	04-Sep-1843	M	first child
Piccioli	Mrs. G.	2159	20-Jul-1852	M	fifth child
Piccioli	Mrs. G.	2715	17-Feb-1856	F	attended by Dr O'Neill
Piccoli	Mrs.	1389	03-Feb-1847	M	third child
Piccoli	Mrs.	1792	27-Dec-1849	F	fourth child
Piccoli	Mrs. A.	1127	14-Feb-1845	M	second child
Pichon	Mrs. Oules	2911	06-Jun-1857	M	first child, forceps delivery
Pickerell	Mrs. J. F.	3338	08-Feb-1860	F	sixth child
Pickerell	Mrs. J. H.	3032	03-Jan-1858	F	fifth child
Pickrell	Mrs.	1438	23-May-1847	F	first child
Pickrell	Mrs. J. F.	1775	19-Nov-1849	M	third child
Pickrell	Mrs. J. F.	2508	09-Nov-1854	F	fourth child
Pickrell	Mrs. J. F.	3521	15-May-1861	M	seventh child
Pickrell	Mrs. J. F.	3749	20-Feb-1863	M	third child
Pickrell	Mrs. J. F.	3891	24-May-1864	F	ninth pregnancy
Pickrell	Mrs. V.	1597	01-Jul-1848	M	second child
Pierce	Mrs. W. H.	3718	18-Dec-1862	F	fifth child
Pierce	Mrs. Wm. H.	4021	22-Aug-1865	M	sixth pregnancy
Pinkney	Mrs. Frederick	772	25-Oct-1842	M	first child
Pinkney	Mrs. Frederick	1154	19-May-1845	F	second child
Pinkney	Mrs. Frederick	1326	01-Sep-1846	F	third child
Pinkney	Mrs. Frederick	2350	08-Nov-1853	F	born 5: 50 AM
Pisani	Mrs. Antoni	3869	21-Mar-1864	M	first pregnancy
Pittering	Mrs. E.	3476	15-Jan-1861	F	second child
Pittman	Mrs. Edward	2980	10-Oct-1857	M	first child
Pittman	Mrs. Edward	3392	10-Jul-1860	F	second child

Obstetrical Casebooks of Dr. F. E. Chatard – an alternative genealogical resource 1829-1883

Pitts	Mrs. Charles	1143	28-Apr-1845		M	first child
Pitts	Mrs. Charles	1456	28-Jul-1847		F	second child
Pitts	Mrs. Charles	1651	03-Dec-1848		M	third child
Pitts	Mrs. Charles	1822	22-Feb-1850		M	fourth child
Pitts	Mrs. Charles A.	2416	28-Apr-1854		M	seventh child
Pitts	Mrs. Charles H.	2188	07-Oct-1852		F	sixth child
Pitts	Mrs. Sullivan	4911	24-Jun-1874		F	first pregnancy
Pitts	Mrs. Sullivan	4984	10-Jun-1875		F	second pregnancy
Pitts	Mrs. Thomas G.	990	08-May-1844		M	second child
Pitts	Mrs. Thomas G.	1251	17-Jan-1846		M	third child
Pitts	Mrs. Thomas G.	712	03-May-1842		M	first child
Placide	Mrs.	539	30-Oct-1840		M	second child
Placide	Mrs.	905	17-Oct-1843		F	third child
Pleasants	. Mrs. Hall	3951	30-Nov-1864		F	third pregnancy
Pleasants	Mrs. Hall	4151	10-Oct-1866		F	fourth pregnancy
Pleasants	Mrs. Hall	4494	22-Oct-1869		M	fifth pregnancy
Pleasants	Mrs. J. Hall	3777	05-May-1863		M	second child
Plummer	Mrs. James	3443	18-Nov-1860		M	first child
Plummer	Mrs. J. W.	4375	09-Oct-1868		M	second pregnancy
Plummer	Mrs. W. J.	3661	28-Jul-1862		F	second child
Plummer	Mrs. W. J.	4778	09-Sep-1872		M	fifth pregnancy
Plummer	Mrs. W. J.	5072	31-Jul-1876		F	sixth pregnancy
Plummer	Mrs. Wm. J.	4099	29-Apr-1866		F	third pregnancy
Plummer	Mrs. Wm. J.	4457	08-Jun-1869		F	fourth pregnancy
Plummer	Mrs. Wm. James	5158	20-May-1878		M	seventh pregnancy

163

Obstetrical Casebooks of Dr. F. E. Chatard – an alternative genealogical resource 1829-1883

Plunkett	Mrs. Henry	2190	15-Oct-1852	F	second child
Poester	Mrs.	1554	20-Mar-1848	M	first child
Polk	Mrs.	84	28-Sep-1833	F	fifth child
Polkinhorn	Mrs. H.	435	10-Nov-1839	F	first child
Polster	Mrs. F.	2919	18-Jun-1857	F	seventh child
Pontier	Mrs. E. F.	2637	16-Aug-1855	F	third child
Pontier	Mrs. Rebecca	1828	20-Mar-1850	M	first child
Poor	Mrs. Alfred	4240	11-Aug-1867	F	eighth pregnancy
Poor	Mrs. Alfred	4466	09-Jul-1869	F	ninth pregnancy
Poor	Mrs. Alfred	4651	16-Apr-1871	M	ninth pregnancy
Poor	Mrs. R.	4613	02-Dec-1870	M	third pregnancy
Poor	Mrs. R. L.	4298	26-Jan-1868	F	second pregnancy
Pope	Mrs. W. H.	5110	23-Mar-1877	M	third pregnancy
Pope	Mrs. Wm.	4837	03-Jun-1873	M	first pregnancy
Pope	Mrs. Wm.	4949	05-Nov-1874	F	second pregnancy
Poppelein	Mrs. George J.	4628	28-Dec-1870	M	first pregnancy, forceps delivery
Popplein	Mrs. George J.	5058	15-Jun-1876	M	second pregnancy, forceps delivery. "It appeared quite healthy when born but two days after its birth it became generally jaundiced and died on the third day."
Portis	Mrs. David	2865	21-Feb-1857	M	fourth child
Portis	Mrs. David	3238	23-May-1859	M	sixth child
Portis	Mrs. David	4076	24-Jan-1866	F	eighth pregnancy
Post	Mrs. W. E.	5100	27-Jan-1877	F	first pregnancy
Post	Mrs. W. E.	5166	20-Aug-1878	F	second pregnancy." The lady resided in Baltimore County & when I arrived I found she had been delivered by Dr Pier of Towsontown."
Postely	Mrs.	260	27-Sep-1837	F	second child

Obstetrical Casebooks of Dr. F. E. Chatard – an alternative genealogical resource 1829-1883

Potts	Mrs.	1572	02-May-1848	M	third child
Poulson	Mrs. A.	377	06-Apr-1839	M	fourth child
Poulson	Mrs. A. W.	627	19-Aug-1841	F	fifth child
Poulson	Mrs. A. W.	994	14-May-1844	F	sixth child
Poulson	Mrs. A. W.	1516	21-Dec-1847	M	first child
Poulson	Mrs. A. W.	1773	12-Nov-1849	F	second child
Poulson	Mrs. A. W.	2382	17-Jan-1854	F	second child
Poulson	Mrs. A. W.	2796	24-Sep-1856	F	fourth child
Poultney	Mrs. Thomas	2039	17-Oct-1851	M	first child
Poultney	Mrs. Thomas	2291	07-Jun-1853	M	second child
Poultney	Mrs. Thomas	2876	12-Mar-1857	M	third child
Powell	Mrs.	2215	05-Dec-1852	M	seventh child
Powell	Mrs. Elizabeth	4450	18-May-1869	M	second pregnancy
Powell	Mrs. R. M.	4697	07-Oct-1871	F	third pregnancy
Powell	Mrs. Robert	3267	06-Sep-1859	F	first child, attended by Dr. Caskey, stillborn
Power	Mrs. E. V.	3784	16-Jun-1863	F	fourth pregnancy
Power	Mrs. John	2912	07-Jun-1857	F	third child
Powers	Mrs. John	2405	19-Mar-1854	M	first child
Powers	Mrs. John	2666	05-Oct-1855	F	second child
Pratt	Mrs.	1010	03-Jul-1844	M	first child, stillborn
Pratt	Mrs.	1222	04-Nov-1845	F	second child
Pratt	Mrs.	1731	25-Jul-1849	F	third child
Pratt	Mrs. H.	467	09-Mar-1840	M	born 7:20 PM
Pratt	Mrs. Wm.	2095	31-Jan-1852	M	fourth child
Pregrans	Mrs.	3356	24-Mar-1860	F	five months pregnant
Prentiss	Mrs. John	3265	23-Aug-1859	M	first child

Obstetrical Casebooks of Dr. F. E. Chatard – an alternative genealogical resource 1829-1883

Preston	Mrs. J. A.	4173	04-Jan-1867	M	third pregnancy
Preston	Mrs. J. Alexander	3882	22-Apr-1864	F	second pregnancy
Preston	Mrs. J. Alexander	4442	26-Apr-1869	M	fourth pregnancy
Preston	Mrs. John	4511	06-Dec-1869	F	first pregnancy
Preston	Mrs. John	4794	05-Nov-1872	M	third pregnancy
Preston	Mrs. John F.	4658	03-May-1871	M	second pregnancy
Preston	Mrs. John F.	4951	10-Nov-1874	F	fourth pregnancy
Preston	Mrs. John F.	5238	06-Jul-1881	F	fifth pregnancy, forceps delivery
Preston, Jr.	Mrs. Jacob A.	3580	01-Nov-1861	M	first child
Prevat	Mrs.	687	22-Feb-1842	F	tenth child
Prevost	Mrs Aristide	3488	09-Feb-1861	M	fifth child
Prevost	Mrs.	417	09-Sep-1839	M	ninth child
Prevost	Mrs. A.	1748	16-Sep-1849	M	13th child
Prevost	Mrs. Aristide	2111	11-Mar-1852	F	second child
Prevost	Mrs. Aristide	2807	14-Oct-1856	F	second child
Prevost	Mrs. Aristide	3055	11-Mar-1858	M	third child
Prevost	Mrs. Aristide	3281	12-Oct-1859	M	fourth child
Prevost	Mrs. Aristide	3679	11-Sep-1862	F	sixth child
Prevost	Mrs. Constance	2631	11-Aug-1855	M	first child
Prevost	Mrs. E.	2590	02-May-1855	F	first child
Prevost	Mrs. Emryale [?]	2852	13-Jan-1857	F	fourth child
Prevost	Mrs. Eurial	3140	04-Oct-1858	M	fourth child
Prevost	Mrs. Euryale	3824	25-Nov-1863	F	fifth pregnancy

Obstetrical Casebooks of Dr. F. E. Chatard – an alternative genealogical resource 1829-1883

Prevost	Mrs. Euryale	4024	29-Aug-1865	F	seventh pregnancy
Prevost	Mrs. Euryale	4346	27-Jun-1868	F	seventh pregnancy
Prevost	Mrs. Euryale	4537	19-Apr-1870	M	eighth pregnancy
Prevost	Mrs. L. Euryole	3579	29-Oct-1861	F	sixth child
Prevost	Mrs. Victor	1840	07-May-1850	M	second child
Prevost	Mrs. Victor	2079	31-Dec-1851	F	third child
Prevost	Mrs. Victor	2387	29-Jan-1854	M	fourth child
Prevost	Mrs. Victor	2704	27-Jan-1856	M	fifth child
Prevost	Mrs. Victor	3095	13-Jun-1858	F	fifth child
Prevost	Mrs. Victor	3331	25-Jan-1860	F	eighth child
Prevot	Madame	1331	09-Sep-1846	F	
Prevot	Mrs.	999	10-Jun-1844	M	11th child
Prevot	Mrs. Victor	1588	23-Jun-1848	M	first child
Price	Mrs.	912	29-Oct-1843	F	first child
Price	Mrs. Alfred	3731	05-Jan-1863	F	colored, third child
Price	Mrs. Alfred	4183	30-Jan-1867	F/F	colored, fifth pregnancy
Price	Mrs. Alfred C.	3945	15-Nov-1864	M	colored, fourth pregnancy
Price	Mrs. Anthony	2535	04-Jan-1855	M	first child
Price	Mrs. B.	4661	11-May-1871	F	first pregnancy
Price	Mrs. Benjamin	4787	13-Oct-1872	M	second pregnancy
Price	Mrs. Doctor	848	15-May-1843		first child, mother convulsed
Price	Mrs. Frances	2169	27-Aug-1852	M	colored, first child
Price	Mrs. George R.	3859	20-Feb-1864	F	third pregnancy
Price	Mrs. Joseph	4064	23-Dec-1865	F	fourth pregnancy
Price	Mrs. Joseph	4202	22-Mar-1867	M	sixth pregnancy

Obstetrical Casebooks of Dr. F. E. Chatard – an alternative genealogical resource 1829-1883

Price	Mrs. R.	21	12-Jan-1831	M	colored at Center St., ninth child
Price	Mrs. Romeo	78	02-Jul-1833		see 12 Jan 1831 [#21], colored, tenth child, child died
Price	Mrs. Romeo	106	26-May-1834		see 2 Jul 1833 [#78], eleventh child, six months, child dead
Price	Mrs. Romeo	199	09-Aug-1836	M	colored
Prior	Mrs. E. A.	4431	23-Mar-1869	M	first pregnancy
Purden	Mrs.	479	13-Apr-1840	F	fourth child
Pyfer	Mrs. Philip	1126	14-Feb-1845	M	second child
Pyfer	Mrs. Philip	2343	06-Oct-1853	F	fourth child
Pyfer	Mrs. Philip	2695	26-Dec-1855	F	fifth child
Pyfer	Mrs. Philip	3053	09-Mar-1858	F	sixth child
Pyfer	Mrs. Philip H.	1531	17-Jan-1848	F	
Pyfer	Mrs. W. B.	1574	11-May-1848	F	fifth child
Quaid	Mrs. James	2864	20-Feb-1857	M	second child
Quaid	Mrs. James	3179	28-Dec-1858	F	third child
Quaid	Mrs. James	3522	16-May-1861	M	fifth child
Quaid	Mrs. James	3789	05-Jul-1863	F	fifth pregnancy
Quarles	Mrs. John	5136	05-Jul-1877	M	first pregnancy, ninth month "She was attacked with a sort of cholera mortus." Headaches & convulsions, forceps delivery
Quigley	Mrs. Edward	2486	26-Sep-1854	F	fourth child
Quigley	Mrs. James	3031	03-Jan-1858	M	first child
Quigley	Mrs. James	3573	27-Sep-1861	M	second child
Quinn	Mrs.	1	01-Aug-1829	F	third child, the umbilical cord was four feet four inches in length and encircled the child's neck twice
Quinn	Mrs.	26	21-Aug-1831	M	fourth child, nine pounds
Quinn	Mrs.	98	14-Mar-1834	F	see 21 Aug 1831 [#26], fifth child, 9.5 lbs

Obstetrical Casebooks of Dr. F. E. Chatard – an alternative genealogical resource 1829-1883

Quinn	Mrs. Charles	1409	26-Mar-1847	F	first child, forceps
Rabillion	Mrs. Leonce	2938	16-Jul-1857	M	second child
Raborg	Mrs. F.	3646	07-Jun-1862	F	sixth child
Raborg	Mrs. F.	3950	27-Nov-1864	F	sixth pregnancy
Raborg	Mrs. F.	4654	23-Apr-1871	M	seventh pregnancy, child deformed, died within 24 hours
Raborg	Mrs. F. W.	3109	03-Aug-1858	F	fourth child
Rafferty	Mrs. John	5247	17-Feb-1882	F	first pregnancy
Rafferty	Mrs. Patrick	2442	27-Jun-1854	M	first child
Rafferty	Mrs. Patrick	2877	12-Mar-1857	M	second child
Ralston	Mrs. J. H.	4536	06-Apr-1870	M	first pregnancy
Ralston	Mrs. Thomas H.	5125	04-Jun-1877	M	second pregnancy
Randall	Mrs.	1939	29-Jan-1851	M	fourth child
Randall	Mrs. J. K.	2500	20-Oct-1854	M	tenth child
Randall	Mrs. J. K.	2890	18-Apr-1857	F	11th child
Randall	Mrs. J. K.	3293	15-Nov-1859	F	12th child. "very small."
Randall	Mrs. S. H.	2166	11-Aug-1852	M	second child
Randolph	Mrs. J. T.	3157	04-Nov-1858	F	second child
Randolph	Mrs. J. T.	3387	23-Jun-1860	F	third child
Randolph	Mrs. J. T.	3901	04-Jul-1864	F	fifth pregnancy
Randolph	Mrs. J. T.	4177	21-Jan-1867	M	sixth pregnancy
Randolph	Mrs. J. T.	4472	02-Aug-1869	F	seventh pregnancy
Randolph	Mrs. James T.	2914	11-Jun-1857	M	first child
Randolph	Mrs. James T.	3618	01-Mar-1862	F	fourth child
Raphel	Mrs. Ameda	3880	16-Apr-1864	M	first pregnancy
Ratican	Mrs. Edward	2579	06-Apr-1855	M	"...the child being born before I arrived."
Ratican	Mrs. Edward	2930	06-Jul-1857	M	seventh child, 6 1/2 months premature, died

169

Obstetrical Casebooks of Dr. F. E. Chatard – an alternative genealogical resource 1829-1883

Ratican	Mrs. John	2555	06-Feb-1855	M	first child
Raticar [?]	Mrs. Michael	2473	05-Sep-1854	F	first child
Rau	Mrs.	1771	08-Nov-1849	M	second child
Rau	Mrs. J. P.	2030	04-Oct-1851	M	third child
Rau	Mrs. John P.	2477	14-Sep-1854	F	fourth child
Rau	Mrs. John P.	3044	15-Feb-1858	M	fourth child
Read	Mrs. W. G.	444	25-Dec-1839	F	fourth child
Read	Mrs. W. G.	791	12-Dec-1842		miscarriage at three months
Read	Mrs. Wm.	4626	24-Dec-1870	M	second pregnancy
Reckert	Mrs. George	2563	01-Mar-1855	M	first child
Reckert	Mrs. George	3173	12-Dec-1858	F	third child
Reckert	Mrs. George	3423	30-Sep-1860	M	fourth child
Reckert	Mrs. George	3675	29-Aug-1862	F	fifth child
Reed	Mrs.	714	07-May-1842	F	first child
Reese	Mrs. D. G.	1248	10-Jan-1846	M	eighth child
Reese	Mrs. G. D.	732	30-Jun-1842	M	eighth child
Reese	Mrs. Henry O.	4447	14-May-1869	M	first pregnancy
Reese	Mrs. Henry O.	4639	29-Jan-1871	F	second pregnancy, eight months
Reese	Mrs. Henry O.	4814	16-Feb-1873	M	third pregnancy
Reeves	Mrs. Joseph	1123	13-Feb-1845	M	born 2:35 PM
Reich	Mrs. DR. P. H.	5207	13-Nov-1879	F	second pregnancy
Reich	Mrs. Dr. P. H.	5245	25-Jan-1882	F	third pregnancy
Reiche	Mrs. Dr. P. H.	5156	29-Apr-1878	F	first pregnancy, "The Doctor informed me that his wife flooded very freely when about that his wife flooded very freely when about two months pregnant … so that he was under the impression that she had

170

Obstetrical Casebooks of Dr. F. E. Chatard – an alternative genealogical resource 1829-1883

Surname	Name	No.	Date	Sex	Notes
Reid	Mrs. Washington	1087	13-Dec-1844	M	aborted." first child
Reidolph	Mrs.	1329	06-Sep-1846	M	seventh child
Reilly	Mrs.	824	24-Feb-1843	M	first child
Reily	Mrs. A. B.	1212	04-Oct-1845	M	third child
Reindollar	Mrs. J. T.	3147	16-Oct-1858	M	second child
Reinhard	Mrs. M.	4699	11-Oct-1871	F	fifth pregnancy
Reinhard	Mrs. M. E.	4053	01-Nov-1865	M	second pregnancy
Reinhard	Mrs. M. E.	4860	11-Oct-1873	F	sixth pregnancy
Reinhard	Mrs. M. E>	4225	14-Jun-1867	M	third pregnancy
Reinhard	Mrs. M. E>	4408	21-Jan-1869	F	fourth pregnancy
Remare	Mrs. A.	1502	24-Nov-1847	F	sixth child
Remare	Mrs. A.	1804	28-Jan-1850	F	ninth child
Rennert	Mrs. Robert	3647	08-Jun-1862	M	second child, attended by Dr. C. Johnston
Rennick, Jr.	Mrs. Robert	4387	19-Nov-1868	M	second pregnancy
Rennick, Jr.	Mrs. Robert	4964	26-Dec-1874	M	fourth pregnancy
Rennolds	Mrs. H. S.	3821	18-Nov-1863	F	third pregnancy
Renshaw	Mrs. Robert	3354	19-Mar-1860	M	first child
Renwick	Mrs. Frank	5189	08-May-1879	F	first pregnancy
Renwick	Mrs. J. A.	4760	15-Jun-1872	F	ninth pregnancy, "The child was premature and did not linger more than a month."
Renwick	Mrs. Robert	4189	12-Feb-1867	F	first pregnancy
Renwick, Jr.	Mrs. Robert	4547	11-May-1870	F	third pregnancy
Renwick, Jr.	Mrs. Robert	4768	17-Jul-1872	M	fourth pregnancy
Renwick, Jr.	Mrs. Robert	5101	31-Jan-1877	F	sixth pregnancy

Obstetrical Casebooks of Dr. F. E. Chatard – an alternative genealogical resource 1829-1883

Renwick, Jr.	Mrs. Robert	5182	06-Mar-1879	F	seventh pregnancy
Reyburn	Mrs.	387	02-Jun-1839	M	first child
Reyburn	Mrs.	527	01-Oct-1840	F	second child
Reynolds	Mrs.	1390	02-Feb-1847	F	fourth child
Reynolds	Mrs. Dr.	3563	29-Aug-1861	F	second child, weighing nearly 14 pounds. "She was a tall & large woman."
Reynolds	Mrs. J.	4716	07-Dec-1871	M	first pregnancy
Reynolds	Mrs. John E.	4853	06-Sep-1873	F	second pregnancy
Reynolds	Mrs. John E.	5005	21-Sep-1875	M	third pregnancy
Reynolds	Mrs. John E.	5108	12-Mar-1877	F	fourth pregnancy, "The patient suffered from intense irritation of the stomach for several months during the latter part of her pregnancy …I hoped … she would be entirely relieved but on the contrary."
Reynolds	Mrs. Joseph	1323	22-Aug-1846	M	second child
Reynolds	Mrs. Joseph	1727	20-Jul-1849	M	third child
Reynolds	Mrs. Joseph	3172	09-Dec-1858	F	fifth child
Reynolds	Mrs. Joseph	3545	20-Jul-1861	M	sixth child
Reynolds	Mrs. Joseph	3898	24-Jun-1864	F	seventh pregnancy
Reynolds	Mrs. Patrick	5034	22-Jan-1876	M	seventh pregnancy
Reynolds	Mrs. Patrick	5117	18-Apr-1877	F	eighth pregnancy
Reynolds	Mrs. Patrick	5157	09-May-1878	F	ninth pregnancy
Reynolds	Mrs. V. C.	3227	05-May-1859	M	third child, stillborn
Reynolds	Mrs. V. C.	3445	23-Nov-1860	M	fifth child
Reynolds	Mrs. V. C.	3631	30-Apr-1862	F	sixth child, dead
Reynolds	Mrs. V. C.	3776	05-May-1863	F	seventh pregnancy. "It gave but slight signs of life. It appeared much diseased."
Reynolds	Mrs. V. C>	4322	09-Apr-1868	M	ninth pregnancy

Rhett	Mrs. Thomas	2955	02-Sep-1857	F	fourth child
Rhett	Mrs. Thomas	3316	03-Jan-1860	F	fifth child
Rhett	Mrs. Thomas S.	2618	14-Jul-1855	M	third child
Rhodes	Mrs. J.	3110	05-Aug-1858	F	second child
Rial	Mrs. Patrick	1227	12-Nov-1845	F	first child
Rial	Mrs. Patrick	1498	16-Nov-1847	F	second child
Ribney	Mrs. George R.	2540	19-Jan-1855	M	second child
Rice	Mrs.	4229	26-Jun-1867	F	third pregnancy
Rice	Mrs. R.	3959	16-Dec-1864	F	second pregnancy
Richardson	Mrs.	80	03-Aug-1833	M	first child, child dead
Richardson	Mrs.	104	21-May-1834	F	see 3 Aug 1833 [#80], second child, seven months, child dead
Rickert	Mrs. George	2795	23-Sep-1856	M	second child
Riddell	Mrs. Alexander	4063	21-Dec-1865	F	fifth pregnancy, "All her previous gestations have terminated unfortunately, being premature & children stillborn." Child was dead
Ridgely	Mrs. Charles	3643	31-May-1862	F	sixth child
Ridgely	Mrs. Charles	4235	19-Jul-1867	M	eighth pregnancy
Ridgely	Mrs. Charles	4445	02-May-1869	F	ninth pregnancy
Ridgely	Mrs. J. Graham	2428	29-May-1854	M	second child
Ridgely	Mrs. J. L.	4030	12-Sep-1865	F	ninth pregnancy
Ridgely	Mrs. John	3652	28-Jun-1862	F	eighth child
Ridgely	Mrs. John	5140	27-Jul-1877	F	(of Hampton), third pregnancy. "The child physician present."
Ridgely	Mrs. John	5259	28-Sep-1882	M	sixth pregnancy
Ridgely	Mrs. Otho	5177	25-Dec-1878	F	first pregnancy
Ridgely	Mrs. Otho	5226	13-Nov-1880	F	second pregnancy
Ridgely	Mrs. Otho	5258	23-Sep-1882	M	third pregnancy
Ridgley	Mrs. Andrew	4016	19-Jun-1865	F	third pregnancy

Obstetrical Casebooks of Dr. F. E. Chatard – an alternative genealogical resource 1829-1883

Ridgley	Mrs. C.	934	12-Dec-1843	F	first child
Ridgley	Mrs. Charles	2308	19-Jul-1853	M	of Hamble [?], second child
Ridgley	Mrs. Charles	2536	07-Jan-1855	M	third child
Ridgley	Mrs. Charles	2705	30-Jan-1856	M	fourth child
Ridgley	Mrs. Charles	3088	29-May-1858	F	fifth child
Ridgley	Mrs. David	915	31-Oct-1843	M	tenth child
Ridgley	Mrs. Graham	2154	09-Jul-1852	M	first child
Ridgley	Mrs. John	595	16-May-1841	F	fifth child
Ridgley	Mrs. John	4912	25-Jun-1874	F	(of Hampton), first pregnancy
Ridgley	Mrs. John	5028	02-Jan-1876	F	second pregnancy
Rielly	Mrs. Charles	5014	24-Oct-1875	F	first pregnancy
Rielly	Mrs. Edward	1046	07-Oct-1844	F	second child
Rielly	Mrs. James	1466	14-Aug-1847	M	born 1 AM
Rielly	Mrs. Patrick	2737	17-Apr-1856	M	second child
Rielly	Mrs. Patrick	3373	24-May-1860	M	third child
Rielly	Mrs. Patrick	3850	31-Jan-1864	F	"labour rapid & natural."
Rielly	Mrs. Ros	2314	03-Aug-1853	M	first child, difficult birth, stillborn
Riely	Mrs.	1547	28-Feb-1848	M	born 4 AM
Riely	Mrs. A. B.	520	21-Aug-1840	M	first child, difficult delivery
Riely	Mrs. A. B.	767	12-Oct-1842	M	second child
Riely	Mrs. A. B.	1578	19-May-1848	M	fourth child
Riely	Mrs. Ann	1026	23-Aug-1844	M	third child
Rieman	Mrs. Joseph H.	4788	22-Oct-1872	M	fifth pregnancy
Riggs	Mrs. Thomas	3107	31-Jul-1858	F	first child
Riggs	Mrs. Thomas	3433	25-Oct-1860	F	second child
Riggs	Mrs. Thomas	3823	24-Nov-1863	M	third pregnancy, stillborn. "She sank about 4 hours after birth of child."

Obstetrical Casebooks of Dr. F. E. Chatard – an alternative genealogical resource 1829-1883

Rigueun [?]	Mrs. Victor	4642	07-Feb-1871	M	fifth pregnancy
Riley	Mrs. D.	807	08-Jan-1843	F	fourth child
Rinedollar	Mrs. J. T.	2510	11-Nov-1854	M	first child
Ring	Mrs.	1492	18-Oct-1847	F	first child
Ringgold	Mrs. C. Frederick	4404	06-Jan-1869	F	first pregnancy
Ringgold	Mrs. J. P.	3659	16-Jul-1862	F	third child
Ringgold	Mrs. John	2866	22-Feb-1857	M	first child
Ringgold	Mrs. John	3310	25-Dec-1859	F	second child
Ringgold	Mrs. John P.	4077	24-Jan-1866	F	fourth pregnancy
Ringgold	Mrs. John P.	4677	11-Jul-1871	F	fifth pregnancy
Ringgold	Mrs. William	4664	17-May-1871	M	fourth pregnancy
Ringgold	Mrs. William	5097	18-Jan-1877	M	fifth pregnancy
Ringgold	Mrs. Wm.	4389	24-Nov-1868	M	third pregnancy
Ringgold	Mrs. Wm. H.	4154	15-Oct-1866	M	second pregnancy
Ringold	Mrs.	40	12-Jan-1832	F	first child
Rippelmeyer	Mrs. C. H.	1737	11-Aug-1849	M	first child
Rivers	Mrs. Jonathan	3161	08-Nov-1858	M	first child
Rivers	Mrs. Jonathan	3301	07-Dec-1859	M	second child
Roach	Mrs. Edward	3757	10-Mar-1863	F	third pregnancy
Roach	Mrs. Edward	4039	10-Oct-1865	F	fourth pregnancy
Roach	Mrs. Edward	4233	10-Jul-1867	M	fifth pregnancy
Roach	Mrs. O.	4824	24-Mar-1873	M	fourth pregnancy
Roach	Mrs. Orvaulx	4683	01-Aug-1871	M	third pregnancy
Roavenac	Mrs. Christopher	4425	06-Mar-1869	M	third pregnancy

Obstetrical Casebooks of Dr. F. E. Chatard – an alternative genealogical resource 1829-1883

Roberts	Mrs.	1741	08-Sep-1849	F	daughter of Mrs. Reynolds, first child
Roberts	Mrs. Edward	3079	28-Apr-1858	M	second child
Robinson	Mrs.	153	27-Jul-1835		first child, forceps delivery, child dead
Robinson	Mrs. D. A.	528	06-Oct-1840	M	sixth child
Robinson	Mrs. G. W.	2419	07-May-1854	F	71 St. Paul St., second child
Robinson	Mrs. George W.	4215	01-May-1867	M	second pregnancy
Robinson	Mrs. George W.	4421	25-Feb-1869	F	third pregnancy
Robinson	Mrs. George W.	4660	11-May-1871	M	fourth pregnancy
Robinson	Mrs. Jane	304	22-May-1838	M	first child
Robinson	Mrs. W. G.	2999	13-Nov-1857	F	third child
Robinson	Mrs. Wm.	1293	17-Jun-1846	M	colored, first child
Robinson	Mrs. Wm. L.	1904	27-Oct-1850	F	eighth child
Rodenwald	Mrs. Henry	2769	15-Jul-1856	F	first child
Rodewald	Mrs. H.	328	22-Aug-1838	F	born at 8 o'clock
Rodgers	Mrs. P.	4861	12-Oct-1873	M	second pregnancy, "Suffered greatly during her pregnancy ... from ascites." Child stillborn
Rodgers	Mrs. Patrick	4741	21-Mar-1872	M	first pregnancy
Rodgers	Mrs. Patrick	4936	22-Sep-1874	M	third pregnancy
Rodgers	Mrs. Patrick	5029	03-Jan-1876	F	fourth pregnancy
Rogers	Mrs.	1247	09-Jan-1846	M	first child
Rogers	Mrs.	1670	08-Feb-1849	M	second child, a patient of Dr. N. R. Smith
Rogers	Mrs. Evan	2451	24-Jul-1854	F	first child
Rogers	Mrs. Evans	2776	30-Jul-1856	F	second child
Rogers	Mrs. Hugh	1399	02-Mar-1847	M	second child
Rogers	Mrs. Hugh	1769	27-Oct-1849	F	third child

Obstetrical Casebooks of Dr. F. E. Chatard – an alternative genealogical resource 1829-1883

Rogers	Mrs. Hugh	1951	26-Feb-1851	F	fourth child
Rogers	Mrs. J.	176	12-Jan-1836		third child
Rogers	Mrs. J. C.	1962	12-Mar-1851	F	first child
Rogers	Mrs. J. C.	2342	05-Oct-1853	F	second child
Rogers	Mrs. James C.	2941	24-Jul-1857	F	third child
Rogers	Mrs. Joseph	280	11-Feb-1838	M	fifth child
Rogers	Mrs. Joseph	1042	15-Sep-1844	F	child born about 1/4 past 8 PM
Rogers	Mrs. Joseph	1376	08-Jan-1847		born 1 AM
Rogers	Mrs. Joseph	1783	08-Dec-1849	F	born 5:15 AM
Rogers	Mrs. Stanley	3564	01-Sep-1861	F	first child
Rogers	Mrs. Stanley	4333	17-May-1868	F	second pregnancy
Rogers	Mrs. Wm. F.	5131	22-Jun-1877	M	fifth pregnancy
Roleson	Mrs. H.	1161	30-May-1845	M	fifth child, The child was made to breathe with great difficulty, nearly three hours having elapsed before that function was established
Roleson	Mrs. W. H.	576	11-Feb-1841	F	third child in 7th month. Infant died next day
Roleson	Mrs. W. H.	730	28-Jun-1842	F	fourth child
Roleson	Mrs. W. H.	1545	25-Feb-1848	M	sixth child
Roloson	Mrs. W. H.	246	25-Aug-1837	F	first child, Chatard assisted his father Dr. Peter Chatard
Roloson	Mrs. Wm.	374	02-Apr-1839	F	second child
Roloson	Mrs. Wm. H.	2698	01-Jan-1856	M	seventh child
Ronayne	Mrs. J. A.	5162	13-Jul-1878	M/F	first pregnancy, twins
Roney	Mrs. Michael	292	20-Mar-1838	F	second child, still born
Rooke	Mrs. Camillus	3287	28-Oct-1859	F	first child
Rooney	Mrs. Anna	3350	10-Mar-1860	M	first child
Rooney	Mrs. James	2356	17-Nov-1853	M	first child

Obstetrical Casebooks of Dr. F. E. Chatard – an alternative genealogical resource 1829-1883

Root	Mrs. Henry	3601	30-Dec-1861	F	second child
Root	Mrs. Henry	3773	20-Apr-1863	F	third pregnancy
Root	Mrs. Henry	4074	19-Jan-1866	M	fourth pregnancy
Rosel	Mrs.	1831	02-Apr-1850	F	first child
Rosensteel	Mrs. G. T.	1732	27-Jul-1849	M	third child
Rosensteel	Mrs. G. W.	1510	12-Dec-1847	F	second child
Rosensteel	Mrs. J. W.	619	09-Aug-1841	M	seventh child
Rosensteel	Mrs. Joseph	53	05-Sep-1832		second child, eight months
Rosensteel	Mrs. Joseph	101	11-Apr-1834	M	see 5 Sep 1832 [#53], third child
Rosensteel	Mrs. Joseph	163	02-Nov-1835	M	see 11 Apr 1834 [#101], fourth child
Rosensteel	Mrs. Joseph	281	11-Feb-1838	F	fifth child
Rosensteel	Mrs. Joseph	440	21-Nov-1839	M	sixth child
Rosensteel	Mrs. Joseph	844	05-May-1843	M	
Rosensteel	Mrs. Joseph	1666	02-Jan-1849	F	11th child
Rosewell	Mrs.	1560	14-Apr-1848		first child
Ross	Mrs. David	4095	23-Mar-1866	F	second pregnancy
Roundtree	Mrs.	299	24-Apr-1838		first child, still born
Roundtree	Mrs.	419	17-Sep-1839	M	second child
Roundtree	Mrs. John	486	04-May-1840	M	first child, twin boys
Roundtree	Mrs. John	735	11-Jul-1842	F	second child
Rowenac	Mrs. C.	4678	14-Jul-1871	M	fourth pregnancy
Roy	Mrs. George	2369	24-Dec-1853	M	born 10 AM
Royston	Mrs. Joshua	1103	16-Jan-1845	M	fourth child
Runcke	Mrs. A.	429	02-Nov-1839	M	first child

Obstetrical Casebooks of Dr. F. E. Chatard – an alternative genealogical resource 1829-1883

Russell	Mrs. Patrick	3715	16-Dec-1862	F	forceps delivery
Russell	Mrs. Patrick	3861	01-Mar-1864	F	second pregnancy
Rustig	Mrs. S.	4116	12-Jul-1866	F	second pregnancy
Rustig	Mrs. Sedgewick	3978	23-Jan-1865	F	first pregnancy
Ruth	Mrs. John	2472	30-Aug-1854	M	fifth child
Rutherford	Mrs. Joseph	3751	23-Feb-1863	F	second pregnancy
Ruths	Mrs.	976	27-Mar-1844	M	second child
Ruths	Mrs. J. S.	1487	02-Oct-1847	F	third child
Ruths	Mrs. John S.	1794	11-Jan-1850	F	third child
Rutter	Mrs.	555	08-Dec-1840	M	first child
Rutter	Mrs. T.	249	30-Aug-1837	F	13th child
Ryan	Mrs.	52	16-Aug-1832	F	third child, "Had been of feeble health & several times very ill."
Ryan	Mrs. J.	4526	27-Jan-1870	F	fifth pregnancy
Ryan	Mrs. Michael	2267	12-Apr-1853	F	second child
Ryan	Mrs. Michael	2602	30-May-1855	F	third child
Ryan	Mrs. Michael	3165	19-Nov-1858	M	Nr. 65 Harford Avenue, first child
Ryan	Mrs. Michael	3732	13-Jan-1863	F	fourth child
Ryder	Mrs. Michael	1930	25-Dec-1850	M	first child
S.	Mrs.	3577	14-Oct-1861	M	first child
Salmon	Mrs. Hamilton H.	1081	30-Nov-1844	M	first child
Salmon	Mrs. W. L.	2816	25-Oct-1856	M	sixth child
Sanders	Mrs. B. J.	1720	03-Jul-1849	M	first child, stillborn. Mother died 4 July
Sanders	Mrs. Beverly	1431	14-May-1847	F	third child
Sanders	Mrs. Beverly	1823	24-Feb-1850	M	fourth child
Sanders	Mrs. Beverly C.	2454	28-Jul-1854	M	fifth child

Obstetrical Casebooks of Dr. F. E. Chatard – an alternative genealogical resource 1829-1883

Sanders	Mrs. Charles	1214	07-Oct-1845	F	first child, attacked by puerperal fever on 4th day but survived
Sanger	Mrs.	1324	23-Aug-1846	M	first child
Sanler	Mrs. Ernest	3830	20-Dec-1863	M	first pregnancy
Saranz	Mrs. Louis	439	19-Nov-1839	fourth child	
Saranz [?]	Mrs. L.	290	14-Mar-1838	M	third child
Sargent	Mrs.	1627	08-Oct-1848	M	eighth child
Sargent	Mrs. Thomas	1201	06-Sep-1845	F	seventh child
Sargent	Mrs. Thomas B.	1004	19-Jun-1844	F	sixth child
Sarnigait	Mrs. Francois	4415	04-Feb-1869	F	born at 3 AM
Saurret	Mrs. G.	3256	20-Jul-1859	M	third child
Savage	Mrs.	173	29-Dec-1835	F	first child
Savary	Mrs. Eugene	1902	21-Oct-1850	M	first child
Savary	Mrs. Louis	631	06-Sep-1841	F	fifth child, mother hysterical; see 19 Nov 1839
Savary	Mrs. Louis	942	14-Jan-1844	F	sixth child
Sawyer	Mrs. N.	490	13-May-1840	F	fourth child
Schaefer	Mrs. A. C.	1105	18-Jan-1845	M	first child
Schaeffer	Mrs. A. C.	1315	11-Aug-1846	F	second child
Schaeffer	Mrs. A. C.	1687	09-Mar-1849	M	third child
Schaeffer	Mrs. A. C.	1905	28-Oct-1850	M	fourth child
Schaeffer	Mrs. A. C.	2260	29-Mar-1853	M	fifth child
Schaeffer	Mrs. A. C.	2615	06-Jul-1855	F	sixth child
Schaffer	Mrs. Adolphus C.	5150	27-Sep-1877	F	first pregnancy
Schamberger	Mrs. Henry	4307	13-Feb-1868	M	first pregnancy

180

Obstetrical Casebooks of Dr. F. E. Chatard – an alternative genealogical resource 1829-1883

Scheck	Mrs. Joseph	770	22-Oct-1842	F	first child
Scheer	Mrs. V.	3736	15-Jan-1863	F	first child
Scheffe	Mrs.	2132	04-May-1852	M	first child, mother died 5th or 6th day
Scheib	Mrs.	284	22-Feb-1838		attended by midwife & Drs. Hintze & Maguire. Died.
Schenck	Mrs. Edwin	4698	10-Oct-1871	M	first pregnancy
Schenck	Mrs. Edwin	4876	02-Jan-1874	M	second pregnancy
Schenck	Mrs. Edwin	4974	29-Mar-1875	F	third pregnancy
Schenck	Mrs. Edwin	5215	10-Feb-1880	M	fourth pregnancy
Schick	Mrs. Joseph	813	20-Jan-1843	F	born 11:30 PM
Schmidt	Mrs. Henry	3783	15-Jun-1863	F	first pregnancy
Schmidt	Mrs. Henry	3948	24-Nov-1864	M	second pregnancy
Schmidt	Mrs. Henry	4197	25-Feb-1867	F	third pregnancy
Schmidt	Mrs. Henry D.	4448	14-May-1869	F	fourth pregnancy
Schmidt	Mrs. Henry D.	4709	27-Nov-1871	M	fifth pregnancy
Schmidt	Mrs. Henry D.	4857	26-Sep-1873	F	sixth pregnancy
Schmidt	Mrs. Henry D.	5010	10-Oct-1875	F	seventh pregnancy
Schmidt	Mrs. Henry D.	5235	01-Apr-1881	M	eighth pregnancy
Schmidt	Mrs. Philip	2556	10-Feb-1855	M	second child
Schmidt	Mrs. Philip	2765	06-Jul-1856	M	third child
Schmidt	Mrs. Phillip	2328	30-Aug-1853	F	first child
Schmidt	Mrs. Phillip	3008	26-Nov-1857	F	fourth child
Schmidt	Mrs. Phillip	4156	31-Oct-1866	F	fifth pregnancy
Schmidt	Mrs. Phillip	4312	07-Mar-1868	M	sixth pregnancy, seven month, "It was very feeble & lived about 10 days."
Schmidt	Mrs. V.	231	24-Apr-1837	F	second child

Surname	First	ID	Date	Sex	Notes
Schmidt	Mrs. V.	399	25-Jul-1839	M	third child
Schmidt	Mrs. V.	734	08-Jul-1842	M	fourth child
Schmidt	Mrs. William	3474	06-Jan-1861	F	third child
Schmidt	Mrs. William	3743	28-Jan-1863	M	fourth child
Schmidt	Mrs. William J.	3065	05-Apr-1858	F	first child
Schmidt	Mrs. Wm.	2047	26-Oct-1851	M	second child
Schmidt	Mrs. Wm.	3243	30-May-1859	M	second child
Schmidt	Mrs. Wm.	4175	13-Jan-1867	M	sixth pregnancy, child stillborn
Schultz	Mrs.	968	13-Mar-1844	M	second child
Schultz	Mrs.	1275	28-Apr-1846	M	third child
Schwartze	Mrs.	400	31-Jul-1839	M	fourth child, all previous children dead
Scott	Mrs.	2859	08-Feb-1857	F	second child
Scott	Mrs. Henry	2802	07-Oct-1856	F	second child
Scott	Mrs. Henry	3576	05-Oct-1861	M	fourth child
Scott	Mrs. Henry C.	2541	19-Jan-1855	M	first child
Scott	Mrs. Henry C.	3408	22-Aug-1860	M	third child
Scott	Mrs. Job	3366	14-May-1860	M	fourth child
Scott	Mrs. Job	3537	25-Jan-1861	F	fifth child
Scott	Mrs. Job	3737	18-Jan-1863	F	sixth child
Scott	Mrs. Job	3889	18-May-1864	M	seventh pregnancy
Scott	Mrs. Job	4190	13-Feb-1867	M	eighth pregnancy
Scott	Mrs. Job	4308	25-Feb-1868	F	ninth pregnancy, child did not survive
Scott	Mrs. Job	4461	26-Jun-1869	F	tenth pregnancy
Scott	Mrs. Job A.	3106	29-Jul-1858	F	third child
Scott	Mrs. T. P.	649	25-Oct-1841	F	fifth child
Scotti	Mrs. L.	198	08-Aug-1836	M	The child was born when I arrived

Obstetrical Casebooks of Dr. F. E. Chatard – an alternative genealogical resource 1829-1883

Scully	Mrs. D.	2680	20-Nov-1855	M	first child
Seaman	Mrs. J. W>	4481	18-Aug-1869	M	fifth pregnancy
Seckken	Mrs.	1719	01-Jul-1849	M	first child
Seeger	Mrs.	799	24-Dec-1842	M	first child
Seeger	Mrs.	1282	19-May-1846	M	second child
Seibill	Mrs. Michael	2904	24-May-1857	M/	seventh child, twins
Seip	Mrs. Robert C.	4338	09-Jun-1868	F	third pregnancy
Selby	Mrs. Almire	1995	27-Jun-1851	F	first child
Selby	Mrs. J. W.	2635	14-Aug-1855	M	third child
Selby	Mrs. John	4054	23-Nov-1865	F	fifth pregnancy
Sellauser	Mrs. R.	3480	25-Jan-1861	M	first child
Sellman	Mrs. J. C.	894	23-Sep-1843	M	sixth child
Semmes	Mrs. R. T.	4717	09-Dec-1871	F	first pregnancy
Seviler	Mrs. J.	1985	10-Jun-1851	M	eighth child
Seymour	Mrs.	3094	10-Jun-1858	M	at St. Vincent's Asylum, first child
Shanberger	Mrs. Henry	4556	28-May-1870	M	second pregnancy
Shanessey	Mrs. James	1019	06-Aug-1844	F	the child was born when I arrived
Shannaman	Mrs.	124	30-Nov-1834	M	see 11 Jan 1833 [#61], fourth child, nine lbs
Shannaman	Mrs.	224	09-Feb-1837	M	fifth child
Shanneman	Mrs.	25	31-Jul-1831	F	second child, cord around child's neck. Both mother & child did well
Shanneman	Mrs.	61	11-Jan-1833	M	see 31 Jul 1831 [#25]; third child; cord twice twisted around neck
Shannessey	Mrs. James	766	04-Oct-1842	M	born 6 PM
Sharkey	Mrs. J.	1148	12-May-1845	M	first child
Shaw	Mrs. J. H.	1817	18-Feb-1850	F	born 8 AM
Shaw	Mrs. W. C.	5217	05-May-1880	M	second pregnancy
Shaw	Mrs. Wm. C.	5169	02-Oct-1878	F	first pregnancy

Obstetrical Casebooks of Dr. F. E. Chatard – an alternative genealogical resource 1829-1883

Shaw	Mrs. Wm. C.	5263	07-Sep-1883	F	third pregnancy
Shea	Mrs. Daniel	4593	02-Oct-1870	M	fifth pregnancy
Shea	Mrs. Thomas	4192	17-Feb-1867	M	first pregnancy
Sheehan	Mrs. Richard	3503	24-Mar-1861	M	second child
Shehan	Mrs. Richard	3283	19-Oct-1859	F	first child
Shelly	Mrs.	853	09-Jun-1843	F	fourth child
Shepherd	Mrs. George	1855	27-Jun-1850	F	born 4 AM
Shepherd	Mrs. Laura	3352	14-Mar-1860	F	first child
Shepherd	Mrs. Wm.	2077	23-Dec-1851	M	first child
Sheppard	Mrs. George	1120	10-Feb-1845	F	fourth child
Sheppard	Mrs. George	1351	03-Nov-1846	F	third child
Shields	Mrs.	1858	04-Jul-1850	M	first child
Shields	Mrs.	2086	21-Jan-1852	M	second child
Shipley	Mrs. J. S.	3009	26-Nov-1857	F	first child
Shock	Mrs. A. H.	3370	18-May-1860	M	sixth child. "The child died in the birth. I did not see her for sometime after."
Shock	Mrs. A. H.	3539	04-Jul-1861	M	seventh child
Shoemaker	Mrs. Saml.	4205	05-Apr-1867	M	seventh pregnancy
Shoemaker	Mrs. Samuel M.	4715	06-Dec-1871	F	ninth pregnancy
Shook	Mrs. A. H.	2336	19-Sep-1853	F	third child
Shook	Mrs. A. H.	2699	06-Jan-1856	M	fourth child
Shook	Mrs. A. H.	4017	08-Jul-1865	M	eighth pregnancy
Shook	Mrs. Albert	2018	22-Aug-1851	M	second child
Shorter	Mrs.	2544	21-Jan-1855	F	fourth child
Shriver	Mrs. Albert	5202	25-Sep-1879	M	sixth pregnancy, "Called to her suddenly in the absence of her physician."

Obstetrical Casebooks of Dr. F. E. Chatard – an alternative genealogical resource 1829-1883

Shriver	Mrs. J. Alexandre	4742	03-Apr-1872	M	eighth pregnancy. "… the seventh son in succession."
Sikken	Mrs. Charles	1972	04-May-1851	M	second child
Simon	Mrs. Adolph	2327	29-Aug-1853	F	first child
Simon	Mrs. Adolph	3129	07-Sep-1858	M	fourth child
Simon	Mrs. Adolph	3720	20-Dec-1862	F	sixth child
Simon	Mrs. Adolphus	2600	25-May-1855	F	second child
Simon	Mrs. Adolphus	2823	13-Nov-1856	F	third child
Simon	Mrs. Adolphus	3444	20-Nov-1860	M	fifth child
Sinclair, Jr.	Mrs. Robert	1388	01-Feb-1847		miscarriage at four months
Sinclair, Jr.	Mrs. Robert	1887	11-Sep-1850	F	ninth child
Sinclair, Jr.	Mrs. R.	1195	20-Aug-1845		premature at three months
Singleton	Mrs. H. L.	4823	22-Mar-1873	F	second pregnancy
Sinnott	Mrs. I.	4866	24-Nov-1873	F	first pregnancy. "The child died early on the 6th December."
Sinnott	Mrs. John	4966	03-Jan-1875	M	second pregnancy
Sirata	Mrs. V.	436	11-Nov-1839	M	premature labor 6 mos, child died
Skinnington	Mrs.	554	05-Dec-1840	M	first child
Skivington	Mrs. D.	3855	06-Feb-1864	F	fourth pregnancy
Skivington	Mrs. David	2927	29-Jun-1857	F	second child
Slagle	Mrs. H.	4126	30-Jul-1866	M	third pregnancy
Slagle	Mrs. Henry C.	3915	01-Aug-1864	F	second pregnancy
Slater	Mrs. George	874	06-Aug-1843	M	born 9 AM
Slater	Mrs. George	1235	07-Dec-1845	F	
Slater	Mrs. George	1590	25-Jun-1848	F	born 9:45 AM
Slater	Mrs. George	1894	27-Sep-1850	F	tenth child

Obstetrical Casebooks of Dr. F. E. Chatard – an alternative genealogical resource 1829-1883

Slater	Mrs. George	2232	19-Jan-1853	F	11th child
Slater	Mrs. George	2780	10-Aug-1856	F	12th child
Slatter	Mrs. Hope H.	509	12-Jul-1840	M	first child, 8.5 pounds
Slatter	Mrs. Hope H.	783	26-Nov-1842	M	second child
Sloan	Mrs. George F.	2478	14-Sep-1854	F	third child
Sloan	Mrs. James	1946	09-Feb-1851	F	second child
Small	Mrs.	110	24-Jun-1834	F	first child, "She had fallen about a fortnight ago, has not felt child for several days." Child dead
Small	Mrs. William	4350	12-Jul-1868	F	first pregnancy
Smith	Mrs. A. C.	833	15-Mar-1843	M	fifth child, mother comatose but recovered, child dead
Smith	Mrs. A. G.	3808	29-Aug-1863	F	second pregnancy
Smith	Mrs. A. W.	2062	25-Nov-1851	M	first child
Smith	Mrs. A. W.	2491	03-Oct-1854	F	third child
Smith	Mrs. A. W.	2745	03-May-1856	F	fourth child
Smith	Mrs. Catherine	2258	18-Mar-1853	F	second child
Smith	Mrs. E. D.	3846	17-Jan-1864	M	first pregnancy
Smith	Mrs. Ellen	3918	15-Aug-1864	F	first pregnancy
Smith	Mrs. H. J.	3597	06-Dec-1861	M	first child
Smith	Mrs. I.	2323	20-Aug-1853	F	fifth child
Smith	Mrs. J. Bayard	3856	08-Feb-1864	F	13th pregnancy
Smith	Mrs. J. C.	2037	13-Oct-1851	M	first child
Smith	Mrs. J. Dean	4075	20-Jan-1866	F	third pregnancy
Smith	Mrs. J. Dean	4330	05-May-1868	F	fourth pregnancy
Smith	Mrs. J. H.	4990	04-Jul-1875	F/F	first pregnancy, called on consultation by Dr. VanBibber. "…violent convulsions preceded by a very severe headache." twins, both dead. Mother died 11 July.

Obstetrical Casebooks of Dr. F. E. Chatard – an alternative genealogical resource 1829-1883

Smith	Mrs. J. Irwin	2669	11-Oct-1855		M	sixth child
Smith	Mrs. J. Irwin	3072	13-Apr-1858		F	seventh child
Smith	Mrs. J. M.	2799	28-Sep-1856		M	nr. 98 S. Exeter St, first child, attended by Dr. Owings.
Smith	Mrs. J. M.	3061	27-Mar-1858		F	second child
Smith	Mrs. J. N.	3961	19-Dec-1864		M	third pregnancy
Smith	Mrs. J. T.	2736	15-Apr-1856		M	fifth child
Smith	Mrs. Job	49	30-Jul-1832			"a case of abortion." 11th child. "Gone about six weeks without any known cause except being much frighted the night before in a dream."
Smith	Mrs. Marshall	3153	30-Oct-1858		M	first child
Smith	Mrs. Marshall P.	3637	18-May-1862		M	second child
Smith	Mrs. Marshall P.	3997	27-Apr-1865		F	third pregnancy
Smith	Mrs. Marshall P.	4296	14-Jan-1868		F	fourth pregnancy
Smith	Mrs. Marshall P.	4464	08-Jul-1869		F	fifth pregnancy
Smith	Mrs. Marshall P.	4727	30-Dec-1871		F	sixth pregnancy
Smith	Mrs. Martin	1485	29-Sep-1847		F	eighth child, attended by Dr. Herman
Smith	Mrs. S.	402	04-Aug-1839		F	breech, died at two hours
Smith	Mrs. Thomas	36	04-Dec-1831		M	fifth child, nine pounds
Smith	Mrs. Thomas	103	07-May-1834		F	child did on the 16th
Smith	Mrs. Wm.	1241	19-Dec-1845		F	first child
Smith	Mrs. Wm.	1550	07-Mar-1848		F	second child
Smith	Mrs. Wm.	1832	04-Apr-1850		F	third child

Obstetrical Casebooks of Dr. F. E. Chatard – an alternative genealogical resource 1829-1883

Surname	Wife	No.	Date	Sex	Notes
Smith	Mrs. Wm.	2103	19-Feb-1852	F	fourth child
Smith	Mrs. Wm.	2352	11-Nov-1853	M	fifth child
Smith	Mrs. Wm.	2611	01-Jul-1855	M	sixth child
Smith, Jr	Mrs. Job	255	11-Sep-1837	F	13th child
Snowden	Mrs. H. W.	4436	28-Mar-1869	F	first pregnancy
Snowden	Mrs. John	3326	17-Jan-1860	M	second child
Snowden	Mrs. Thoams	4453	19-May-1869	F	tenth pregnancy
Snowdon	Mrs. J. T.	3739	22-Jan-1863	M	eighth child
Sokken	Mrs. Charles	2275	03-May-1853	M	third child
Sokken	Mrs. Charles	3184	17-Jan-1859	F	fifth child
Soper	Mrs. S. J.	3665	07-Aug-1862	M	first child
Soper	Mrs. Samuel	4455	21-May-1869	F	third pregnancy
Soper	Mrs. Samuel J.	3902	04-Jul-1864	F	second pregnancy
Spalding	Mrs.	508	07-Jul-1840	F	second child
Spalding	Mrs. B. R.	238	05-Jun-1837	F	second child
Spalding	Mrs. Wm.	3299	03-Dec-1859	M	eighth child
Spear	Mrs. Edward	4816	24-Feb-1873	M	second pregnancy
Spear	Mrs. Edward W.	4571	13-Jul-1870		first pregnancy, forceps delivery & chloroform
Speckelesen	Mrs. G. A.	1129	15-Feb-1845	M	born 5:10 AM
Spence	Mrs. Carroll	1061	21-Oct-1844	F	first child
Spence	Mrs. Carroll	1606	31-Jul-1848	M	third child
Spencer	Mrs.	416	08-Sep-1839	M	first child
Spencer	Mrs.	644	18-Oct-1841	F	second child
Spencer	Mrs. Carroll	1319	16-Aug-1846	F	second child
Spencer	Mrs. Jervis	4018	09-Jul-1865	M	first pregnancy, forceps delivery

188

Obstetrical Casebooks of Dr. F. E. Chatard – an alternative genealogical resource 1829-1883

Spencer	Mrs. W. H.	3249	20-Jun-1859	F	second child
Spencer	Mrs. W. H.	3554	12-Aug-1861	F	third child
Spencer	Mrs. Wm. H.	2974	08-Oct-1857	M	first child, forceps delivery
Spicer	Mrs. Francis	4043	24-Oct-1865	M	first pregnancy. "She had several convulsions throughout the day and became quite unconscious … she did not recover her consciousness until the morning of 26th."
Spies	Mrs.	579	15-Mar-1841	M	first child
Spies	Mrs.	1267	23-Mar-1846	M	third child
Spies	Mrs. C.	870	25-Jul-1843	F	second child
Spies	Mrs. C.	1592	29-Jun-1848	M	fourth child
Spies	Mrs. C. L.	2089	24-Jan-1852	F	sixth child
Spies	Mrs. C. L.	2501	21-Oct-1854	M	seventh child
Spies	Mrs. C. S.	1762	15-Oct-1849	M	fifth child
Spies	Mrs. Charles	3262	11-Aug-1859	M	"… occurred during my absence."
Spilcker	Mrs. C. W.	1238	11-Dec-1845	M	She was attacked by puerperal fever and died on the 10th day
Spileker	Mrs. C. W.	940	30-Dec-1843	F	third child
Spilker	Mrs.	393	19-Jun-1839	F	second child
Spilker	Mrs.	652	02-Nov-1841	M	third child
Spiller	Mrs. R.	4944	19-Oct-1874	M	third pregnancy
Spiller	Mrs. R. M.	4877	17-Jan-1874	F	second pregnancy
Spilman	Mrs.	37	25-Dec-1831	F	fourth month of pregnancy, fourth child, child died
Spilman	Mrs. P.	2706	01-Feb-1856	M	fourth child
Spretzel	Mrs.	2233	20-Jan-1853	M	second child
Spriggs	Mrs. Emily	2583	13-Apr-1855	F	third child
Spurrier	Mrs. N.	288	13-Mar-1838	M	second child
Spurrier	Mrs. Nelson	517	15-Aug-1840	F	third child

Obstetrical Casebooks of Dr. F. E. Chatard – an alternative genealogical resource 1829-1883

Spurrier	Mrs. Nelson	787	05-Dec-1842	F	fourth child
Spurrier	Mrs. Windham	574	03-Feb-1841	F	first child
Spurrier	Mrs. Windham	774	06-Nov-1842	M	second child
Spurzel	Mrs. A.	2578	05-Apr-1855	F	third child
Stagler	Mrs. Mark	4167	10-Dec-1866	F	second pregnancy
Stapleton	Mrs.	405	05-Aug-1839	F	second child
Stapleton	Mrs. Joshua	1180	28-Jul-1845	M	
Stark	Mrs. Capt.	1368	20-Dec-1846	F	third child
Starkey	Mrs. J.	1523	06-Jan-1848	M	third child
Starkey	Mrs. John	1339	23-Sep-1846	F	second child
Starkey	Mrs. John	1781	02-Dec-1849	F	fourth child
Starkey	Mrs. John	1992	24-Jun-1851	M	fifth child
Starkey	Mrs. John	2239	10-Feb-1853	M	sixth child
Starkey	Mrs. John	2487	27-Sep-1854	M	seventh child
Starkey	Mrs. John	2798	28-Sep-1856	F	eighth child
Starkey	Mrs. John	3132	16-Sep-1858	F	ninth child
Starkey	Mrs. John	3399	30-Jul-1860	F	tenth child
Starkey	Mrs. John	3795	28-Jul-1863	F	11th pregnancy
Staub	Mrs. Richard	4465	12-Jul-1869	F	second pregnancy
Staub	Mrs. Richard P.	4722	23-Dec-1871	F	third pregnancy
Staylor	Mrs. George	2256	17-Mar-1853	F	first child
Staylor	Mrs. Henry	3559	24-Aug-1861	M	first child
Staylor	Mrs. Mark	3911	23-Jul-1864	M	first pregnancy, forceps delivery
Steadman	Mrs.	270	26-Nov-1837	M	first child
Steadman	Mrs.	373	30-Mar-1839	F	second child

190

Obstetrical Casebooks of Dr. F. E. Chatard – an alternative genealogical resource 1829-1883

Stechfield	Mrs.	1870	05-Aug-1850	F	fifth child
Stechfield	Mrs.	2395	19-Feb-1854	F	eighth child
Steel	Mrs. J. Nevitt	4035	26-Sep-1865	M	ninth pregnancy
Stein	Mrs. Samuel	5078	20-Aug-1876	F	third pregnancy
Stellman	Mrs. John	1845	24-May-1850		third child
Stellman	Mrs. John	2436	09-Jun-1854	F	fifth child
Stellman	Mrs. John	3056	15-Mar-1858	F	eighth child
Stellman	Mrs. John	3404	04-Aug-1860	M	ninth child
Stellman	Mrs. John	4025	03-Sep-1865	F	12th pregnancy
Stellman	Mrs. John	4282	23-Nov-1867	M	13th pregnancy
Stellman	Mrs. John H.	5095	06-Jan-1877	M	first pregnancy
Stellmann	Mrs. J.	1612	11-Aug-1848	F	third child
Stellmann	Mrs. John	2121	01-Apr-1852	M	fourth child
Stendler	Mrs.	1308	17-Jul-1846	F	born 4:30 AM
Stendler	Mrs. John	1653	07-Dec-1848	F	fifth child
Stendler	Mrs. John	1943	05-Feb-1851	F	sixth child
Stendler	Mrs. John	2376	08-Jan-1854	F	first child
Stephens	Mrs. Josephine	2389	30-Jan-1854	F	first child
Sterling	Mrs. Archibald	2721	09-Mar-1856	M	first child
Stettmann	Mrs. John	2775	30-Jul-1856	F	sixth child
Steuart	Mrs. Charles	1948	18-Feb-1851	F	first child
Steuart	Mrs. Charles	4563	19-Jun-1870	F	second pregnancy
Steuart	Mrs. Dr. James	2568	15-Mar-1855	F	second child
Steuart	Mrs. G. H.	258	14-Sep-1837	F	previous children all boys
Steuart	Mrs. General	1336	21-Sep-1846	F	11th child

191

Obstetrical Casebooks of Dr. F. E. Chatard – an alternative genealogical resource 1829-1883

Steuart	Mrs. George H.	877	14-Aug-1843	F	ninth child
Steuart	Mrs. James	2093	27-Jan-1852	F	first child
Steuart	Mrs. John	2815	24-Oct-1856	M	second child
Steuart	Mrs. R. S.	424	13-Oct-1839	M	ninth child
Steuart	Mrs. W. H.	995	15-May-1844	F	
Steuart	Mrs. W. H.	1740	08-Sep-1849	F	third child, attended by Dr. Baer, child died
Steuart	Mrs. Wm. H.	1404	16-Mar-1847	F	born1 AM
Steuart	Mrs. Wm. H.	1695	28-Mar-1849	M	eighth child
Steudemeyer	Mrs. Jacob	2598	20-May-1855	F	first child, attended by Dr. George Gibson. "It made a few attempts at breathing but died soon after."
Stevens	Mrs.	1014	15-Jul-1844	F	second child
Stevenson	Mrs.	415	07-Sep-1839	M	fourth child
Stevenson	Mrs. G. B.	703	04-Apr-1842	M	fifth child
Stevenson	Mrs. G. B.	1027	24-Aug-1844	M	sixth child
Stevenson	Mrs. George B.	1236	07-Dec-1845	M	sixth child
Stevenson	Mrs. J. M.	2561	24-Feb-1855	M	first child
Stewart	Mrs. Charles M.	3460	09-Dec-1860	F	third child
Stewart	Mrs. Charles M.	5236	07-May-1881	F	tenth pregnancy
Stewart	Mrs. Charles M.	2332	12-Sep-1853	F	second child
Stewart	Mrs. Charles M.	3673	25-Aug-1862	F	fourth child
Stewart	Mrs. Charles M.	4198	02-Mar-1867	F	first pregnancy
Stewart	Mrs. Charles M.	4360	02-Aug-1868	F	second pregnancy
Stewart	Mrs. Charles M.	4544	10-May-1870	M	third pregnancy
Stewart	Mrs. Charles	4656	29-Apr-1871	M/	fourth pregnancy, twins
Stewart	Mrs. D.	211	15-Oct-1836	F	first child

192

Obstetrical Casebooks of Dr. F. E. Chatard – an alternative genealogical resource 1829-1883

Stewart	Mrs. David	339	01-Oct-1838	M	second child
Stewart	Mrs. F. A.	4657	01-May-1871	M	second pregnancy
Stewart	Mrs. F. A.	4478	15-Aug-1869	M	first pregnancy
Stewart	Mrs. J. D.	4574	20-Jul-1870	F	tenth pregnancy
Stewart	Mrs. John	2650	06-Sep-1855	F	third child
Stewart	Mrs. John	3085	25-May-1858	F	third child
Stewart	Mrs. John	3459	09-Dec-1860	F	Nr. 77 Oregon St., first child
Stewart	Mrs. John	3625	16-Apr-1862	F	fourth child
Stewart	Mrs. John D.	4302	02-Feb-1868	F	ninth pregnancy
Stewart	Mrs. Josephine	2453	27-Jul-1854	F	first child
Stewart	Mrs. W.	2019	24-Aug-1851	M	attended by her father, Dr. Baer
Stewart	Mrs. W. H.	2085	20-Jan-1852	F	ninth child, stillborn
Stiford	Mrs.	1473	05-Sep-1847	M	first child
Stiltz	Mrs.	237	30-May-1837	M	seventh child
Stiltz	Mrs.	482	21-Apr-1840	M	difficult birth
Stinchomb	Mrs. George	2793	20-Sep-1856	M	first child
Stinchomb	Mrs. George	3057	15-Mar-1858	F	second child
Stinchomb	Mrs. George	3288	29-Oct-1859	M	third child
Stinchomb	Mrs. George	3595	02-Dec-1861	F	fourth child
Stinchomb	Mrs. George	4134	12-Aug-1866	M	sixth pregnancy
Stirling	Mrs. Murray	3867	18-Mar-1864	F	first pregnancy
Stirling, Jr.	Mrs. Archibald	4085	25-Feb-1866	M	sixth pregnancy
Stock [?]	Mrs. A. H.	3123	29-Aug-1858	M	fifth child
Stoddard	Mrs.	145	14-May-1835	F	first child
Stoker	Mrs. M.	2569	19-Mar-1855	M	second child
Stokes	Mrs. D. W.	543	21-Nov-1840	M	first child

193

Obstetrical Casebooks of Dr. F. E. Chatard – an alternative genealogical resource 1829-1883

Stokes	Mrs. Robert	3068	07-Apr-1858	M	12th child
Stoneman	Mrs. General	4157	04-Nov-1866	F	second pregnancy
Stoneman	Mrs. Genl.	3686	30-Sep-1862	M	first child
Storke	Mrs. A. L.	4972	13-Feb-1875	F	first pregnancy
Storke	Mrs. A. L.	5084	16-Oct-1876	F	second pregnancy
Stout	Mrs. Richard P.	4351	16-Jul-1868	M	first pregnancy, stillborn
Straney	Mrs.	156	02-Aug-1835	M	see Ms. McCadon 23 Apr 1831, [#22], fourth child
Straney	Mrs. Edward	679	30-Jan-1842	F	rapid labor. Child died 5 Feb 1842
Straney	Mrs. John	285	22-Feb-1838	F	fifth child
Straney	Mrs. John	542	16-Nov-1840	F	sixth child
Straney	Mrs. John	967	12-Mar-1844	M	born about 8:30 PM
Stratter	Mrs.	264	05-Oct-1837	M	second child, breech, died in one hour
Stratton	Mrs.	352	28-Nov-1838	M	fourth child
Stratton	Mrs.	775	08-Nov-1842	M	fifth child
Stratton	Mrs. R.	578	04-Mar-1841	F	fourth child
Stratton	Mrs. R.	1287	01-Jun-1846	F	born 4 AM
Stratton	Mrs. R.	1480	18-Sep-1847	F	child born 10:15 PM
Stratton	Mrs. R.	1717	25-Jun-1849	F	born 9 AM
Stratton	Mrs. Richard	2181	22-Sep-1852	M	ninth child, stillborn
Stratton	Mrs. Richard	2474	06-Sep-1854	M	11th child
Strohm	Mrs.	2531	26-Dec-1854	M	14 1/2 S. Calvert St., first child
Strohm	Mrs. H. F.	3254	09-Jul-1859	M	third child
Strohn	Mrs. H. F.	2958	04-Sep-1857	M	second child
Stryker	Mrs. A. P.	4668	07-Jun-1871	F	second pregnancy, consultation with Dr. Van Bibber, forceps delivery. "The child was delivered but life was extinct."
Stuard	Mrs. C. P.	4117	12-Jul-1866	M	first pregnancy

Obstetrical Casebooks of Dr. F. E. Chatard – an alternative genealogical resource 1829-1883

Stuart	Mrs. E. V.	3921	31-Aug-1864	F	first pregnancy
Stump	Mrs.	518	17-Aug-1840	F	third child
Sullivan	Mrs. D.	330	25-Aug-1838	F	second child
Sullivan	Mrs. D.	642	15-Oct-1841	F	third child
Sullivan	Mrs. Daniel N.	5143	20-Aug-1877	F	fifth pregnancy
Sullivan	Mrs. Dennis	1490	11-Oct-1847	F	fifth child
Sullivan	Mrs. Felix	4482	19-Aug-1869	F	first pregnancy
Sullivan	Mrs. Felix	4950	07-Nov-1874	M	third pregnancy
Sullivan	Mrs. Felix	5053	04-May-1876	F	fourth pregnancy
Sullivan	Mrs. Franklin	1359	30-Nov-1846	M	second child
Sullivan	Mrs. H.	456	11-Jan-1840	M	first child
Sullivan	Mrs. H.	1292	15-Jun-1846	M	fourth child
Sullivan	Mrs. H. P.	675	18-Jan-1842	M	second child
Sullivan	Mrs. H. P.	1626	04-Oct-1848	M	fourth child
Sullivan	Mrs. Henry	1969	09-Apr-1851		fourth child
Sullivan	Mrs. J.	4527	03-Feb-1870	F	third pregnancy
Sullivan	Mrs. James	4428	15-Mar-1869	F	first pregnancy
Sullivan	Mrs. John	3705	14-Nov-1862	M	third child
Sullivan	Mrs. P. H.	945	17-Jan-1844	M	third child
Sulski	Mrs.	421	22-Sep-1839	M	third child
Sutro	Mrs. Otto	4587	15-Sep-1870	F	first pregnancy
Sutro	Mrs. Otto	4729	04-Jan-1872	F	second pregnancy
Suullian	Mrs. H.	1508	05-Dec-1847	F	born 1 AM
Swain	Mrs. Jarrett	2182	22-Sep-1852	F	seventh child
Swain	Mrs. Jarrett	2648	04-Sep-1855	F	eighth child

Name	Title	#	Date	Sex	Notes
Swann	Mrs. Thomas	1150	15-May-1845		seventh child, child born before I arrived
Switzer	Mrs.	2581	08-Apr-1855	F	fourth child
Symington	Mrs.	1069	03-Nov-1844	M	child was born before I arrived
Symington	Mrs. Thomas	676	18-Jan-1842	F	born 6 AM
Talbott	Mrs. Thom. E.	1756	28-Sep-1849	F	second child
Taylor	Mrs.	50	13-Aug-1832	M	West Fayette St., third child, "Very delicate." Has been under care of Dr. Potter. "The child died about the 10th day wasting gradually away."
Taylor	Mrs.	86	11-Oct-1833	F	see 13 Aug 1832 [#50], fourth child
Taylor	Mrs.	177	19-Jan-1836	F	see 11 Oct 1833 [#86], fifth child
Taylor	Mrs.	392	19-Jun-1839	F	first child; mother seized and died on 22nd
Taylor	Mrs.	1182	30-Jul-1845	M	first child
Taylor	Mrs. B.	552	04-Dec-1840		assisted Dr. Perkins
Taylor	Mrs. Col.	1714	06-Jun-1849	M	eighth child
Taylor	Mrs. W. H.	2069	10-Dec-1851	M	fourth child
Taylor	Mrs. Winfield J.	5130	22-Jun-1877	F	first pregnancy
Templeman	Mrs. R. W.	3627	20-Apr-1862	F	second child
Templeman	Mrs. R. W.	3805	17-Aug-1863	M	third pregnancy
Templeman	Mrs. R. W.	4199	03-Mar-1867	F	fifth pregnancy
Templeman	Mrs. R. W.	4591	28-Sep-1870	F	sixth pregnancy
Tennant	Mrs. T.	839	17-Apr-1843		miscarriage at three months
Tennant	Mrs. Thomas	1504	28-Nov-1847	F	difficult birth, Mother died on 4 Dec. The child was almost lifeless when born, we however succeeded in causing it to breath
Thelin	Mrs. W.	4702	20-Oct-1871	F	third pregnancy
Thelin	Mrs. William	4625	15-Dec-1870	F	second pregnancy
Thelin	Mrs. William	4831	06-May-1873	M	fourth pregnancy

Obstetrical Casebooks of Dr. F. E. Chatard – an alternative genealogical resource 1829-1883

Theobald	Mrs. Dr.	1163	06-Jun-1845	F		second child
Thomas	Madame Francois	1949	22-Feb-1851	F		fourth child
Thomas	Mrs.	0	11-Dec-1850			fifteen leeches to uterus …
Thomas	Mrs.	236	25-May-1837			fifth child, varicella, child died on 10th day
Thomas	Mrs. D. E.	4462	02-Jul-1869	M		fifth pregnancy
Thomas	Mrs. David E.	4718	09-Dec-1871	F		sixth pregnancy, weight 12 pounds
Thomas	Mrs. Dr. J. H.	906	18-Oct-1843	F		third child
Thomas	Mrs. Francois	2231	19-Jan-1853	M		fifth child
Thomas	Mrs. J. H.	2036	10-Oct-1851	F		seventh child
Thomas	Mrs. J. Harrison	1372	01-Jan-1847	M		fifth child
Thomas	Mrs. J. J.	4743	07-Apr-1872	M		attended by Dr. W. Howard. "the child born with life almost extinct, but was finally brought to & cried freely."
Thomas	Mrs. J.H.	634	21-Sep-1841	M		second child
Thomas	Mrs. John A.	1707	19-May-1849	F		sixth child
Thomas	Mrs. John H.	1048	08-Oct-1844	M		third child
Thomas	Mrs. John H.	3308	20-Dec-1859			fourth child, dead. "She became exceedingly feeble & required brandy, … ammonia & to sustain her. She was exceedingly prostrate for several days & recovered with great difficulty."
Thomas	Mrs. John Hansa	2362	05-Dec-1853	M		eighth child
Thomas	Mrs. Lt.	1451	07-Jul-1847	F		fourth child
Thomas	Mrs. Lt.	1847	27-May-1850	M		fifth child
Thomas	Mrs. Lt.	2100	13-Feb-1852	F		seventh child
Thomas	Mrs. Lt.	2259	22-Mar-1853	F		eighth child

Obstetrical Casebooks of Dr. F. E. Chatard – an alternative genealogical resource 1829-1883

Thomas	Mrs. Philip F.	2000	12-Jul-1851	F	tenth child
Thomas	Mrs. Philip F.	2547	23-Jan-1855	F	12th child
Thomas	Mrs. Philip H.	2211	25-Nov-1852	F	11th child
Thomas	Mrs. Phillip F.	3074	17-Apr-1858	F	13th child
Thomas	Mrs. Philp	4292	27-Dec-1867	M	sixth pregnancy
Thomas	Mrs. Pierre	3232	13-May-1859	M	sixth child
Thomas	Mrs. W.	1782	05-Dec-1849	F/F	ninth child, twins
Thomas	Mrs. W. G.	2294	10-Jun-1853	M	tenth child
Thomas, Jr.	Mrs. David J.	4252	07-Sep-1867	M	forceps delivery
Thompson	Mrs. A. W.	379	25-Apr-1839	F	sixth child
Thompson	Mrs. A. W.	495	29-May-1840	M	seventh child
Thompson	Mrs. A. W.	722	29-May-1842	M	eighth child
Thompson	Mrs. A. W.	1000	11-Jun-1844	F	seventh child
Thompson	Mrs. A. W.	1330	07-Sep-1846	M	ninth child
Thompson	Mrs. A. W.	1610	05-Aug-1848	F	11th child
Thompson	Mrs. D. B>	4486	30-Aug-1869	M	first pregnancy
Thompson	Mrs. D. Bowly	4842	29-Jun-1873	M	third pregnancy, difficult birth, mother died 2 July
Thompson	Mrs. G. C.	2881	17-Mar-1857	M	second child
Thompson	Mrs. G. C.	3239	24-May-1859	M	third child
Thompson	Mrs. George C.	2526	15-Dec-1854	M	first child. "The child gave no signs of life."
Thompson	Mrs. Joseph B.	2565	10-Mar-1855	F	fifth child
Thompson	Mrs. Joseph B.	3199	20-Feb-1859	F	sixth child
Thompson	Mrs. S.	636	22-Sep-1841	F	second child
Thompson	Mrs. S. T.	345	01-Nov-1838	F	third child
Thompson	Mrs. S. T.	922	21-Nov-1843	F	sixth child
Thompson	Mrs. Stephen	880	22-Aug-1843	F	sixth child

Obstetrical Casebooks of Dr. F. E. Chatard – an alternative genealogical resource 1829-1883

Thomson	Mrs. J. J.	4871	24-Dec-1873	F	fifth pregnancy
Thurner, Jr.	Mrs. J.	4459	20-Jun-1869	F	second pregnancy
Tiernan	Mrs. Charles	1054	17-Oct-1844	F	born 5:30 AM
Tiffany	Mrs. George P.	2726	16-Mar-1856	F	first child
Tiffany	Mrs. George P.	3188	22-Jan-1859	M	second child
Tiffany	Mrs. Henry	1049	10-Oct-1844	M	third child
Tiffany	Mrs. Osmond	1918	21-Nov-1850	F	second child
Tiffany	Mrs. William S.	3007	25-Nov-1857	M	first child
Tiffany, Jr	Mrs. Osmond	1661	09-Jan-1849	M	first child
Tiffany, Jr.	Mrs. Osmond	2193	23-Oct-1852	M	third child
Tileston	Mrs.	132	06-Jan-1835	F	second child, "The child had a good deal of difficulty in swallowing which disappeared only when she began to take the breast."
Tilghman	Mrs. Capt. R.	3648	12-Jun-1862	F	eighth child
Tilghman	Mrs. Lloyd	1204	14-Sep-1845	M	second child
Tilghman	Mrs. Lloyd	1519	29-Dec-1847	M	third child
Tilghmann	Mrs. Lt. N.	2653	10-Sep-1855	F	sixth child
Tilghmann	Mrs. Richard	1770	29-Oct-1849	F	third child
Tinges	Mrs. G. M.	1521	01-Jan-1848	F	child born 9 AM
Tinges	Mrs. G. W.	2493	06-Oct-1854	F	seventh child
Tinges	Mrs. G. W.	2872	04-Mar-1857	F	eighth child
Tinges	Mrs. George W.	2157	15-Jul-1852	M	sixth child
Tinges	Mrs. George W.	3162	17-Nov-1858	M	ninth child
Toldridge	Mrs. W. H.	3543	16-Jul-1861	F	second child
Tolts	Mrs.	924	26-Nov-1843	M	attended by Dr. Maguire, forceps delivery
Tolts	Mrs.	1171	01-Jul-1845	M	second child
Tomkins	Mrs. E.	1025	20-Aug-1844	M	first child

Obstetrical Casebooks of Dr. F. E. Chatard – an alternative genealogical resource 1829-1883

Tonge	Mrs. G. W.	1837	25-Apr-1850	M	fifth child
Tonry	Mrs. William P.	5090	08-Nov-1876	F	fourth pregnancy
Tonry	Mrs. Wm. P.	4535	31-Mar-1870	M	first pregnancy
Tonry	Mrs. Wm. P.	5187	24-Apr-1879	F	fifth pregnancy
Tormey	Mrs. E. J.	4003	11-May-1865	M	first pregnancy
Tormey	Mrs. E. J.	4129	05-Aug-1866	F	second pregnancy
Torney	Mrs. G.	4792	01-Nov-1872	M	first pregnancy
Torney	Mrs. George H.	5030	06-Jan-1876	F	second pregnancy
Torwy [?]	Mrs. Wm. P.	4988	02-Jul-1875	M	third pregnancy
Towson	Mrs. C.	1002	16-Jun-1844	F	premature, six months
Towson	Mrs. Charles	1194	19-Aug-1845	F	seventh child
Towson	Mrs. Charles	1548	04-Mar-1848	F	born 12 AM, stillborn
Towson	Mrs. Charles	1856	27-Jun-1850	F	tenth child
Trail	Mrs. F. M.	1166	14-Jun-1845	M	second child
Trail	Mrs. R. H.	3078	28-Apr-1858	F	first child
Trail	Mrs. R. H.	3593	22-Nov-1861	F	second child
Trail	Mrs. R. H.	3771	20-Apr-1863	M	third pregnancy. "Although constantly stimulated … sunk & died on the 5th day."
Trainer	Mrs. B.	349	06-Nov-1838	F	first child
Trainer	Mrs. Barney	512	25-Jul-1840	M	second child
Trainer	Mrs. Bernard	1321	13-Aug-1846	M	attended by my father [Dr. Peter Chatard].
Trainer	Mrs. Bernard	1520	25-Dec-1847		The child was born some time before I saw her
Trainer	Mrs. Bernard	1833	09-Apr-1850	F	eighth child
Trainer	Mrs. Bernard	2107	01-Mar-1852	F	ninth child
Trainer	Mrs. Bernard	2604	30-May-1855	F	tenth child

200

Obstetrical Casebooks of Dr. F. E. Chatard – an alternative genealogical resource 1829-1883

Trainer	Mrs. Bernard	2758	08-Jun-1856	F	11th child
Trainer	Mrs. J.	4275	02-Nov-1867	M	second pregnancy
Trainer	Mrs. J.	4458	18-Jun-1869	M	third pregnancy
Trainer	Mrs. James	4093	21-Mar-1866	F	first pregnancy
Treadway	Mrs. Henry A.	1683	03-Mar-1849	M	first child
Treadwell	Mrs.	406	07-Aug-1839	F	third child
Treadwell	Mrs.	1169	23-Jun-1845	F	sixth child
Treadwell	Mrs. O. W.	603	25-Jun-1841	M	fourth child, forceps delivery
Treadwell	Mrs. O. W.	830	09-Mar-1843	M	fifth child, 11 1/2 pounds
Treadwell	Mrs. O. W.	1511	12-Dec-1847	F	seventh child
Trider	Mrs.	2855	25-Jan-1857	M	fifth child
Trillard	Mrs. August	4977	14-Apr-1875	F	second pregnancy
Trundle	Mrs. W. B.	4864	31-Oct-1873	M	first pregnancy
Truss	Mrs. Nelson	4040	11-Oct-1865	F	first pregnancy
Tubman	Mrs. B. G.	3169	05-Dec-1858	M	second child
Tucker	Mrs. H. R.	876	11-Aug-1843	M	first child
Tucker	Mrs. H. R.	1055	17-Oct-1844	F	second child
Tucker	Mrs. H. R.	1302	01-Jul-1846	M	third child
Tucker	Mrs. H. R.	1555	20-Mar-1848	M	fourth child
Tucker	Mrs. Henry R.	1865	29-Jul-1850	M	fifth child
Tucker	Mrs. Wesley	4492	16-Oct-1869	M	sixth pregnancy
Tufts	Mrs. Wm.	275	31-Dec-1837	M	third child
Turnbull	Mrs. A. N.	4669	09-Jun-1871	F	third pregnancy
Turnbull	Mrs. A. N.	5040	18-Feb-1876	F	fifth pregnancy
Turnbull	Mrs. A. Nesbit	4517	23-Dec-1869		second pregnancy, stillborn

Obstetrical Casebooks of Dr. F. E. Chatard – an alternative genealogical resource 1829-1883

Turnbull	Mrs. A. Nesbit	4836	25-May-1873	M	fourth pregnancy
Turnbull	Mrs. H.	657	23-Nov-1841	M	third child, 11 pounds
Turnbull	Mrs. Henry	372	14-Mar-1839	M	first child
Turnbull	Mrs. Henry	842	27-Apr-1843	M	fourth child
Turnbull	Mrs. Henry	1036	05-Sep-1844	F	fifth child
Turnbull	Mrs. Henry	1332	11-Sep-1846	M	sixth child
Turnbull	Mrs. Henry	1601	13-Jul-1848	M	seventh child
Turnbull	Mrs. Henry	1818	19-Feb-1850	M	eighth child
Turnbull	Mrs. Henry	2094	29-Jan-1852	M	ninth child
Turnbull	Mrs. J. Lisle	4484	28-Aug-1869	F	first pregnancy, forceps delivery
Turnbull	Mrs. J. Lisle	4707	21-Nov-1871	M	second pregnancy
Turnbull	Mrs. J. Lisle	4867	02-Dec-1873	M	third pregnancy, headache, blurred vision & swelling "She was put on use of Gettysburg Spring water." The child was dead
Turnbull	Mrs. Laurence	4711	29-Nov-1871	M	firth pregnancy, "The labour was slow & painful."
Turnbull	Mrs. Nesbit	4413	01-Feb-1869	F	first pregnancy
Turner	[-?-]	357	01-Jan-1839	M	a colored woman belonging to Miss Claggett, first
Turner	Anney	190	15-Jun-1836		see 9 Feb 1834 [#96], third child
Turner	Mrs. Calhoun	1119	09-Feb-1845	F	seventh child
Turner	Mrs. Calhoun	1377	08-Jan-1847	M	eight child
Turner	Mrs. Catherine	1643	13-Nov-1848	M	ninth child. About an hour & a half after birth of child, she had some hemorrhage & great prostration which was controlled by ice, vinegar & Brandy
Turner	Mrs. J. E.		07-Oct-1845		miscarriage at three months
Turner	Mrs. J. E.	1645	15-Nov-1848		third child, stillborn
Turner	Mrs. J. H.	3389	30-Jun-1860	F	sixth child

Obstetrical Casebooks of Dr. F. E. Chatard – an alternative genealogical resource 1829-1883

Turner	Mrs. J. H.	3619	03-Mar-1862	M	seventh child, 7 months. "It lived but a few hours."
Turner	Mrs. James	3710	01-Dec-1862	M	first child
Turner	Mrs. Richard	1211	02-Oct-1845	M	
Turner	Mrs. Richard	1373	02-Jan-1847	M	third child
Turner	Mrs. Richard	1577	14-May-1848	F	fourth child
Turner	Mrs. Richard	2053	09-Nov-1851	M	fifth child
Turner	Mrs. S. E.	1328	06-Sep-1846	M	first child
Turner	Mrs. S. E.	2196	24-Oct-1852	F	fifth child
Turner	Mrs. Samuel E.	1836	21-Apr-1850	M	fifth child, premature 6 months
Turner	Mrs. W. F.	1976	12-May-1851	M	tenth child
Turner, Jr.	Mr. J. T.	4870	23-Dec-1873	M	fourth pregnancy
Turner, Jr.	Mrs. J. J.	4378	17-Oct-1868	M	first pregnancy
Turner, Jr.	Mrs. J. J.	4583	06-Sep-1870	F	second pregnancy
Turner, Jr.	Mrs. J. J.	4754	15-May-1872	F	third pregnancy
Turner, Jr.	Mrs. John	4325	16-Apr-1868	F	attended by Dr. Gough, first pregnancy
Turner, Jr.	Mrs. Joseph J.	5082	30-Sep-1876	F	sixth pregnancy
Tyson	Mrs. A. H.	1140	14-Apr-1845	M	the child was born a little after 12 before I arrived at her residence 10 miles in the country
Tyson	Mrs. J. E.	2124	21-Apr-1852	F	second child
Tyson	Mrs. James N.	2505	26-Oct-1854	F	third child
Tyson	Mrs. James W.	4487	26-Sep-1869	M	ninth pregnancy, attended by Dr. J. Cary Thomas, stillborn
Tyson	Mrs. Julia	2492	05-Oct-1854	F	first child
Tyson	Mrs. Richard	2720	08-Mar-1856	M	second child
Vacara	Mrs. Antonio	2528	18-Dec-1854	F	second child
Valentine	Mrs.	1767	26-Oct-1849	M	seventh child

Obstetrical Casebooks of Dr. F. E. Chatard – an alternative genealogical resource 1829-1883

Valette	Mrs. Victor	1353	11-Nov-1846		The child having been born when I arrived
Valette	Mrs. Victor	1677	16-Feb-1849	M	tenth child
Valetti	Mrs. Victor	771	23-Oct-1842	M	seventh child
Vallance	Mrs. W. H.	3669	13-Aug-1862	F	fourth child, eight months
Van Derwater	Mrs. J.	4598	17-Oct-1870	M	eighth pregnancy. "The child was born about 10 AM. It cried feebly & made some attempt to breath but all my efforts to save it were in vain."
Van Ness	Mrs. Col. E.	3052	08-Mar-1858	M	eighth child
Van Ness	Mrs. Eugene	4355	24-Jul-1868	M	first pregnancy
Van Ness	Mrs. Eugene	4605	01-Nov-1870	M	second pregnancy
Van Ness	Mrs. Eugene	4913	05-Jul-1874	M	third pregnancy
Van Schalkenich	Mrs Adrien	4184	01-Feb-1867	F	second pregnancy
VanKapff	Mrs. H.	3992	12-Apr-1865	M	fifth pregnancy
VanKapff	Mrs. Henry	4221	25-May-1867	F	sixth pregnancy
VanKapff	Mrs. Herman	3211	16-Mar-1859	M	second child
Vanlill	Mrs. Stephen	1897	06-Oct-1850	F	first child
Vansant	Mrs.	324	16-Aug-1838	F	fourth child
Vansant	Mrs. R.	239	12-Jun-1837		miscarriage at 6 months
Vansant	Mrs. R.	476	02-Apr-1840	F	first child
Vaughan	Mrs. Henry	4397	27-Dec-1868	M	first pregnancy
Vickers	Mrs. A.	2817	25-Oct-1856	M	sixth child
Vickers	Mrs. Albert	711	23-Apr-1842	M	first child
Vickers	Mrs. Albert	939	29-Dec-1843	F	born 7 AM
Vickers	Mrs. Albert	2140	26-May-1852	M	born 1:20 AM
Vickers	Mrs. B. A.	1419	09-Apr-1847	M	third child
Vickers	Mrs. B. A.	1667	01-Feb-1849	F	fourth child

Obstetrical Casebooks of Dr. F. E. Chatard – an alternative genealogical resource 1829-1883

Vickers	Mrs. B. A.	3210	16-Mar-1859	M	seventh child
Vickers	Mrs. Frank	5105	18-Feb-1877	M	first pregnancy
Vickers, Jr.	Mrs. George R.	5112	27-Mar-1877	F	second pregnancy, attended by Dr. Schmidt
Volz	Mrs.	635	22-Sep-1841	M	second child
Volz	Mrs. P.	430	03-Nov-1839	M	first child
Volz	Mrs. Peter	1272	15-Apr-1846	F	fourth child
Volz	Mrs. Peter	1624	02-Oct-1848	M	fifth child
Volz	Mrs. Peter	1881	30-Aug-1850	F	sixth child
Volz	Mrs. Peter	2335	18-Sep-1853	F	seventh child
Volz	Mrs. Peter	2756	05-Jun-1856	M	eighth child
Volz	Mrs. Peter	3248	20-Jun-1859	F	ninth child
von Bokkeller	Mrs. Libertus	2994	10-Nov-1857	F	third child
VonKaff	Mrs. F.	1678	18-Feb-1849	M	second child
VonKaff	Mrs. Frederick	2377	08-Jan-1854	M	third child
VonKaff	Mrs. J.	1375	07-Jan-1847	M	first child
VonKapff	Mrs. Frederick	2729	25-Mar-1856	F	fourth child
VonKapff	Mrs. H.	3424	30-Sep-1860	M	third child
VonKapff	Mrs. Herman	2902	15-May-1857	F	first child
VonKapff	Mrs. Herman	3707	19-Nov-1862	M	fourth child
VonKapff	Mrs. Herman	4485	28-Aug-1869	M	seventh pregnancy
Voss	Mrs. B. F.	888	07-Sep-1843	F	seventh child
Voss	Mrs. B. F.	1591	28-Jun-1848	M	ninth child
Voss	Mrs. B. F.	1886	11-Sep-1850	F	tenth child
Voss	Mrs. F.	412	02-Sep-1839	F	fourth child
Voss	Mrs. Franklin	604	29-Jun-1841	M	sixth child

Obstetrical Casebooks of Dr. F. E. Chatard – an alternative genealogical resource 1829-1883

Voss	Mrs. Franklin	1223	05-Nov-1845	F	
Wagner	Mrs. Basil	5049	04-Apr-1876	F	first pregnancy
Wagner	Mrs. Basil	5120	05-May-1877	M	second pregnancy
Wagner	Mrs. Basil	5192	05-Jun-1879	M	third pregnancy
Wagner	Mrs. Basil	5231	17-Jan-1881	F	fourth pregnancy
Wagner	Mrs. Charles J.	4429	15-Mar-1869	F	first pregnancy
Walker	Mrs. J.	371	12-Mar-1839	F	a colored woman, first child
Walker	Mrs. J.	498	13-Jun-1840	M	colored woman (see #371), second child
Walker	Mrs. W. J.	3515	02-May-1861	M	first child
Wall	Mrs. J.	3493	19-Feb-1861	M	fourth child
Wallack	Mrs. A.	1024	18-Aug-1844	F	second child
Walsh	Mrs.	1984	10-Jun-1851	M	third child
Walsh	Mrs. W. B.	2463	16-Aug-1854	M	fifth child
Walsh	Mrs. Wm. B.	2225	26-Dec-1852	F	fourth child
Walter	Mrs. G. W.	2345	14-Oct-1853	M	fourth child
Walter	Mrs. George	989	04-May-1844	F	second child, breech
Walter	Mrs. George W.	2131	03-May-1852	M	third child
Walters	Mrs.	1385	28-Jan-1847	M	first child
Walters	Mrs. J.	4550	22-May-1870	F	sixth pregnancy
Walters	Mrs. W. J.	2269	18-Apr-1853	F	third child
Walters	Mrs. Wm. F.	1621	26-Sep-1848	M	second child
Walther	Mrs. Peter	3790	12-Jul-1863	F	second pregnancy
Walther	Mrs. Peter	4060	10-Dec-1865	M	third pregnancy
Wampler	Mrs.	13	03-May-1830	M	second child
Wamsley	Mrs. J. S.	4901	09-May-1874	F	second pregnancy

206

Obstetrical Casebooks of Dr. F. E. Chatard – an alternative genealogical resource 1829-1883

Wamsley	Mrs. J. S.	4980	14-May-1875	M	third pregnancy
Wamsley	Mrs. John	4585	09-Sep-1870	M	second pregnancy
Ward	Mrs.	5			residing near Govanstown, attended in the first instances by my father
Ward	Mrs.	30	14-Oct-1831	M	residing near Govanstown, seven months, child died
Ward	Mrs.	511	22-Jul-1840	F	second child
Ward	Mrs.	2293	09-Jun-1853	F	first child
Ward	Mrs.	4166	10-Dec-1866	M	first pregnancy
Ward	Mrs. B.	4009	28-May-1865	M	first pregnancy, forceps delivery
Ward	Mrs. Bernard	4270	26-Oct-1867	F	second pregnancy
Ward	Mrs. David	2773	22-Jul-1856	M	second child
Ward	Mrs. F. X.	4469	22-Jul-1869	F	first pregnancy, six months, child dead
Ward	Mrs. F. X.	4635	16-Jan-1871	M	third pregnancy, six months, mother lost sight, she died 28 Feb 1871
Ward	Mrs. G. W.	1018	01-Aug-1844	M	third child
Ward	Mrs. Hugh	4203	26-Mar-1867	M	first pregnancy
Ward	Mrs. J.	2779	09-Aug-1856	F	third child
Ward	Mrs. James	4137	19-Aug-1866	M	third pregnancy
Ward	Mrs. James	4500	05-Nov-1869	F	fifth pregnancy
Ward	Mrs. Patrick	2623	22-Jul-1855	M	first child
Ward	Mrs. W.	1360	01-Dec-1846	F	fourth child
Ward	Mrs. W.	1673	13-Feb-1849	F	born 10 PM
Ward	Mrs. W.	3036	20-Jan-1858	F	(Dugan), first child
Ward	Mrs. Washington	1772	11-Nov-1849	M	sixth child
Ward	Mrs. Washington	2076	19-Dec-1851	F	seventh child

207

Obstetrical Casebooks of Dr. F. E. Chatard – an alternative genealogical resource 1829-1883

Ward	Mrs. Wm.	1899	15-Oct-1850	F		tenth child
Ward	Mrs. Wm.	3336	04-Feb-1860	F		second child
Ward	Mrs. Wm.	3906	18-Jul-1864	M		first pregnancy
Ward	Mrs. Wm. J.	2909	04-Jun-1857	M		third child
Ward	Mrs. Wm. T.	2484	22-Sep-1854	M		first child
Warden	Mrs. Jesse	385	14-May-1839	M		fourth child
Warder	Mrs. George	2446	17-Jul-1854	F		seventh child, "It died the following night."
Warder	Mrs. George A.	2548	26-Jan-1855			premature five months
Warder	Mrs. George T.	2738	18-Apr-1856	F		third child. Mother died on the 21st.
Wardwell	Mrs.	4620	10-Dec-1870	M		second pregnancy, attended by Dr. Gibson
Warfield	Mrs.	845	09-May-1843	M		second child
Warfield	Mrs. A.	958	07-Feb-1844	F		first child
Warfield	Mrs. A.	1325	28-Aug-1846			second child, deformed
Warfield	Mrs. A.	1481	22-Sep-1847	M		third child
Warfield	Mrs. A.	2016	18-Aug-1851	F		premature 8 months
Warfield	Mrs. A.	2657	20-Sep-1855	F		sixth child
Warfield	Mrs. Daniel	3103	26-Jul-1858	M		second child
Warfield	Mrs. Wm.	596	23-May-1841	M		first child. Mother had headache
Warfield	Mrs. Wm.	1246	04-Jan-1846	F		third child
Warfield, Jr.	Mrs. D.	2725	13-Mar-1856	M		first child
Warm	Mrs. James	896	26-Sep-1843	F		fifth child
Warner	Mrs. Dr.	2573	25-Mar-1855	M		third child
Warner	Mrs. Franklin	3441	08-Nov-1860	F		second child
Warren	Mrs.	778	13-Nov-1842	M		first child
Warrington	Mrs.	169	21-Dec-1835			abortion of nine weeks

208

Obstetrical Casebooks of Dr. F. E. Chatard – an alternative genealogical resource 1829-1883

Washburn	Mrs.	1697	29-Mar-1849	M	first child
Washburn	Mrs. W. F.	2735	09-Apr-1855	M	third child
Washburn	Mrs. W. F.	3738	19-Jan-1863	M	fifth child
Washburn	Mrs. W. T.	2250	24-Feb-1853	F	second child
Washburn	Mrs. Wyman F.	3475	13-Jan-1861	M	fourth child
Waters	Mrs. John	5141	30-Jul-1877	M	fifth pregnancy
Waters	Mrs. R. N.	4162	30-Nov-1866		first pregnancy, attended by Dr. A. Dubin
Waterson	Mrs.	160	16-Oct-1835	M	aged 37, first child, forceps delivery, "quite a stout boy."
Waterson	Mrs.	274	28-Dec-1837	F	second child
Watkins	Mrs.		21-Jul-1840		miscarriage at three months
Watkins	Mrs. George	1774	16-Nov-1849	F	seventh child, stillborn
Watkins	Mrs. George R.	4361	06-Aug-1868	M	first pregnancy
Watklins	Mary	2031	05-Oct-1851	F	colored. First child
Watters	Mrs.	2950	20-Aug-1857	F	first child
Watters	Mrs. F. J.	3547	24-Jul-1861	M	third child
Watters	Mrs. Lt.	3253	05-Jul-1859	M	second child
Watters	Mrs. Lt. J.	3797	31-Jul-1863	F	fourth pregnancy
Watters	Mrs. Wm. J. H.	4507	02-Dec-1869	M	first pregnancy, attended by Dr. W. C. VanBibber, child dead
Weatherby	Mrs. J.	3687	09-Oct-1862	F	fourth child
Weatherby	Mrs. J.	3397	23-Jul-1860	M	third child
Weatherly	Mrs. Maria	2469	27-Aug-1854	F	first child
Weatherly	Mrs. Maria	2709	06-Feb-1856	F	second child
Weaver	Mrs. A. Ward	3985	24-Mar-1865	F	first pregnancy
Webb	Mrs. George	266	02-Nov-1837	M	second child, a boy of large size
Webster	Mrs. C. H.	3812	26-Sep-1863	M	first pregnancy

Obstetrical Casebooks of Dr. F. E. Chatard – an alternative genealogical resource 1829-1883

Weir	Mrs. Robert	4830	02-Apr-1873	F	first pregnancy
Weir	Mrs. Robert	4993	02-Aug-1875	F	second pregnancy, forceps delivery
Weir	Mrs. Robert	5151	28-Sep-1877	F	third pregnancy
Weld	Mrs. Arthur	2538	13-Jan-1855	F	first child
Weld	Mrs. Arthur T.	4181	25-Jan-1867	F	attended by Dr. VanBibber
Wells	Mrs.	350	19-Nov-1838	F	first child
Wells	Mrs. A. W.	669	08-Jan-1842	M	third child, severe hemorrhage
Wells	Mrs. E. A.	2192	18-Oct-1852	F	fifth child
Wells	Mrs. John	1229	18-Nov-1845	M	second child
Welsh	Mrs.	113	25-Jul-1834	F	"The child was expelled before I arrived."
Welsh	Mrs. J.	710	20-Apr-1842	F	fifth child
Welsh	Mrs. J.	1178	13-Jul-1845	F	sixth child
Welsh	Mrs. J.	1517	23-Dec-1847	F	seventh child
West	Mrs. J. T.	4893	28-Mar-1874	F	second pregnancy
Whealey	Mrs.	3663	06-Aug-1862	F	fourth child
Whedbee	Mrs. J. S.	4921	15-Aug-1874	M	first pregnancy
Whedbee	Mrs. J. S.	5161	01-Jul-1878	M	third pregnancy
Whedbee	Mrs. J. S.	5208	18-Nov-1879	M	fourth pregnancy
Whedbee	Mrs. J. S.	5246	05-Feb-1882	M	fifth pregnancy
Whedbee	Mrs. James S.	5063	29-Jun-1876	M	second pregnancy
Wheeden	Mrs. J. H.	3142	06-Oct-1858	M	first child
Wheeler	Mrs.	58	23-Nov-1832	M	sixth child, "very tedious labor."
Wheeler	Mrs. Clement	2676	03-Nov-1855	M	first child
Wheeler	Mrs. David	232	29-Apr-1837	F	second child
Wheeler	Mrs. David	496	02-Jun-1840	F	third child
Wheeler	Mrs. David	916	01-Nov-1843	F	fifth child

Obstetrical Casebooks of Dr. F. E. Chatard – an alternative genealogical resource 1829-1883

Wheeler	Mrs. David	1250	10-Jan-1846	M	born before 1 AM
Wheeler	Mrs. David	1580	20-May-1848	M	first pregnancy
Wheeler	Mrs. J.	4885	08-Feb-1874	F	first child
Wheeler	Mrs. J. D.	151	05-Jul-1835	M	fourth child
Wheeler	Mrs. J. David	680	30-Jan-1842	F	sixth child
Wheeler	Mrs. T. M.	1413	02-Apr-1847	F	third child
Wheelock	Mrs.	2688	12-Dec-1855	F	first child
Wheelock	Mrs. A.	1872	05-Aug-1850	M	second child
Wheelwright	Mrs.	1350	02-Nov-1846	F	first child
Wheelwright	Mrs. J.	1080	29-Nov-1844	F	fourth child
Wheelwright	Mrs. Jesse	3006	24-Nov-1857	F	first child
Whelan	Mrs. Thomas	941	08-Jan-1844	M	third child
Whelan	Mrs. Thomas	2499	14-Oct-1854	M	fourth child
Whelan	Mrs. Thomas	2800	01-Oct-1856	F	fifth child
Whelan	Mrs. Thomas	3371	19-May-1860	F	second child
Whelan	Mrs. William	367	25-Feb-1839	M	fourth child
Whelan	Mrs. Wm.	835	22-Mar-1843	F	first child
White	Mrs.	100	01-Apr-1834		first child
White	Mrs.	836	30-Mar-1843	F	first pregnancy, attended by Dr. Stevenson, forceps delivery
White	Mrs. A. A.	4784	01-Oct-1872	M	third child
White	Mrs. C. R.	1750	18-Sep-1849	M	11th pregnancy
White	Mrs. Charles R.	3781	05-Jun-1863	F	second child
White	Mrs. Charles R.	1570	28-Apr-1848	M	fourth child
White	Mrs. Charles R.	1926	13-Dec-1850	F	Nr. 178 Mulberry St. second pregnancy
White	Mrs. J.	4696	01-Oct-1871	F	

211

Obstetrical Casebooks of Dr. F. E. Chatard – an alternative genealogical resource 1829-1883

White	Mrs. J. C.	586	13-Apr-1841	M	first child
White	Mrs. J. C.	893	21-Sep-1843	F	third child
White	Mrs. J. C.	2270	19-Apr-1853	M	11th child
White	Mrs. J. C.	2449	22-Jul-1854	F	12th child
White	Mrs. J. C.	2629	09-Aug-1855	M	13th child
White	Mrs. J. Campbell	1075	18-Nov-1844	M	fourth child
White	Mrs. J. Campbell	1232	01-Dec-1845	F	fifth child
White	Mrs. J. Campbell	1513	17-Dec-1847	M	seventh child
White	Mrs. J. Campbell	1688	11-Mar-1849	M	eighth child
White	Mrs. John	3422	30-Sep-1860	F	first child
White	Mrs. John	4105	26-May-1866	M	second pregnancy
White	Mrs. John	1369	24-Dec-1846	F	sixth child
White	Mrs. John	2843	15-Dec-1856	F	14th child
White	Mrs. John J.	4437	29-Mar-1869	F	first pregnancy
White	Mrs. John J.	4976	10-Apr-1875	M	third pregnancy
White	Mrs. Wm.	218	05-Jan-1837	M	second child
Whiteby	Mrs.	3400	30-Jul-1860	F	third child
Whiteford	Mrs. J. A.	2074	15-Dec-1851	M	premature, sixth child, stillborn
Whiteford	Mrs. James	2186	03-Oct-1852	F	born 12 midnight
Whiting	Mrs. Rosa	2333	13-Sep-1853	M	first child
Whitridge	Mrs. H.	1188	04-Aug-1845	F	second child
Whitridge	Mrs. H.	1512	15-Dec-1847	F	third child

Obstetrical Casebooks of Dr. F. E. Chatard – an alternative genealogical resource 1829-1883

Whitridge	Mrs. H.	1724	13-Jul-1849	M	fourth child
Whitridge	Mrs. H.	2001	15-Jul-1851	F	fifth child
Whitridge	Mrs. H.	2304	09-Jul-1853	M	sixth child
Whitridge	Mrs. H.	3540	06-Jul-1861	M	eighth child
Whitridge	Mrs. Horatio	2937	14-Jul-1857	F	seventh child
Wight	Mrs. J. J.	2933	08-Jul-1857	M	sixth child
Wight	Mrs. J. J.	3213	19-Mar-1859	M	seventh child
Wight	Mrs. John	1854	27-Jun-1850	M	sixth child
Wight	Mrs. John J.	2084	19-Jan-1852	F	fourth child
Wight	Mrs. John. J.	2437	13-Jun-1854	M	fifth child
Wight	Mrs. O.	1584	02-Jun-1848	M	third child
Wight	Mrs. O. B.	1988	17-Jun-1851	M	fourth child
Wight	Mrs. O. B.	2163	01-Aug-1852	M	fifth child
Wight	Mrs. O. B.	2824	14-Nov-1856	F	seventh child
Wight	Mrs. O. B.	3202	27-Feb-1859	F	eighth child
Wight	Mrs. Oliver	1220	25-Oct-1845	F	first child
Wight	Mrs. Oliver	1382	20-Jan-1847	M	second child
Wigman	Mrs. C.	1009	27-Jun-1844	F	first child
Wilby	Mrs. A. B.	3461	10-Dec-1860	F	first child. "I could not remain in attendance & requested Dr. G. Gibson to be sent for."
Wilcox	Hanson J.	3025	26-Dec-1857	F	second child
Wilcox	Mrs. J. H.	1271	06-Apr-1846	F	second child, It breathed with great difficulty and was brought to by a prolonged warm bath, friction and the interval … use of brandy
Wilcox	Mrs. John	993	12-May-1844	M	first child
Wilcox	Mrs. John H.	1879	23-Aug-1850	F	third child
Wilcox	Mrs. John H.	2830	23-Nov-1856	M	sixth child

Obstetrical Casebooks of Dr. F. E. Chatard – an alternative genealogical resource 1829-1883

Wilcox	Mrs. John H.	3112	09-Aug-1858	M	sixth child
Wilkins	Mrs. Dr. John	4496	25-Oct-1869	F	third pregnancy
Wilkins	Mrs. E. M.	4208	18-Apr-1867	F	first pregnancy
Wilkins	Mrs. Henry	1090	23-Dec-1844	M	first child
Wilkinson	Mrs.	46	07-May-1832	F	first child, six pounds
Wilkinson	Mrs.	99	23-Mar-1834	M	see 7 May 1832 [#46], second child, 6.25 lbs
Wilkinson	Mrs. Charlotte J.	1183	02-Aug-1845	M	fourth child
Wilkinson	Mrs. W.	4112	30-Jun-1866	M	second pregnancy
Wilkinson	Mrs. W. S.	3654	04-Jul-1862	M	first child
Wilkinson	Mrs. Walter	4427	15-Mar-1869	F	third pregnancy
Willen	Mrs. J. W.	3279	07-Oct-1859	M	second child
Williams	Julia	529	11-Oct-1840	M	colored, first child
Williams	Mary	2849	27-Dec-1856	M	colored, first child, attended by Dr Rider, stillborn
Williams	Mrs.	27-Jun-1833	No delivery. She passed a blood clot		
Williams	Mrs.	785	01-Dec-1842	F	from North Carolina, first child
Williams	Mrs. B. H.	3591	16-Nov-1861	F	second child
Williams	Mrs. Dr. W. P.	2671	25-Oct-1855	F	third child
Williams	Mrs. George	2749	17-May-1856	F	fourth child
Williams	Mrs. George	3440	07-Nov-1860	F	a little over 8 months pregnant
Williams	Mrs. George A.	2151	29-Jun-1852	F	second child
Williams	Mrs. George A.	2455	01-Aug-1854	F	third child
Williams	Mrs. George A.	4143	04-Sep-1866	F	sixth pregnancy
Williams	Mrs. George P.	2767	13-Jul-1856	F	third child

Obstetrical Casebooks of Dr. F. E. Chatard – an alternative genealogical resource 1829-1883

Williams	Mrs. H.	2316	05-Aug-1853	M	first child, forceps birth
Williams	Mrs. J.	3763	01-Apr-1863	M	second child
Williams	Mrs. J.	4059	08-Dec-1865	F	third pregnancy
Williams	Mrs. J.	4565	22-Jun-1870	F	fourth pregnancy
Williams	Mrs. J. Savage	5066	13-Jul-1876	F	fourth pregnancy
Williams	Mrs. Jackson A.	3442	16-Nov-1860	M	first child
Williams	Mrs. John A.	5036	28-Jan-1876	F	fifth pregnancy
Williams	Mrs. L. F.	5115	04-Apr-1877	M	fourth pregnancy
Williams	Mrs. N.	1441	04-Jun-1847	M	first child
Willin	Mrs. Joseph E.	3644	02-Jun-1862	M	11th child
Wills	Mrs. W.	4560	16-Jun-1870	M	second pregnancy
Wills	Mrs. W. G.	3320	10-Jan-1860	M	second child
Wills	Mrs. W. H.	4998	24-Aug-1875	F	fifth pregnancy
Wills	Mrs. Wm. H.	5138	14-Jul-1877	M/	sixth pregnancy, twins: 9.25 lbs & 8.5 lbs
Wilmer	Mrs. Pere	4975	06-Apr-1875	F	second pregnancy
Wilmer	Mrs. Pere	5060	23-Jun-1876	F	third pregnancy
Wilmer	Mrs. Pere	5154	01-Apr-1878	M	fourth pregnancy
Wilnor	Mrs.	2162	28-Jul-1852	M	first child
Wilsom	Mrs. Wm.	1052	15-Oct-1844	M	
Wilson	, Sarah	3091	02-Jun-1858	F	colored, seventh child
Wilson	Mrs.	170	22-Dec-1835	M	first child
Wilson	Mrs.	828	03-Mar-1843	M	colored, fourth child
Wilson	Mrs. Charles	3004	17-Nov-1857	M	second child
Wilson	Mrs. D. S.	442	06-Dec-1839	M	second child, nine years after first
Wilson	Mrs. Dr.	1463	11-Aug-1847	F	second child

215

Obstetrical Casebooks of Dr. F. E. Chatard – an alternative genealogical resource 1829-1883

Wilson	Mrs. Franklin	2033	07-Oct-1851		M	first child
Wilson	Mrs. Franklin	2587	25-Apr-1855		M	second child
Wilson	Mrs. George H.	5122	16-May-1877		M	first pregnancy, forceps delivery
Wilson	Mrs. Henry	1615	17-Sep-1848		M	first child
Wilson	Mrs. Henry	1780	28-Nov-1849		M	second child
Wilson	Mrs. Henry	2155	12-Jul-1852		F	third child
Wilson	Mrs. Henry R.	2506	06-Nov-1854		F	fourth child
Wilson	Mrs. J. L. N.	2732	06-Apr-1856		M	second child
Wilson	Mrs. James	1882	31-Aug-1850		M	colored, second child
Wilson	Mrs. James	2137	25-May-1852		M	colored, third child
Wilson	Mrs. James	2289	04-Jun-1853		M	colored, fourth child
Wilson	Mrs. James	2553	01-Feb-1855		M	colored, fifth child
Wilson	Mrs. James	2731	03-Apr-1856		M	colored, sixth child
Wilson	Mrs. James	3598	14-Dec-1861		M	colored, ninth child
Wilson	Mrs. John	3583	08-Nov-1861		F	nr. 28 Holliday St., first child. "Some hours after confinement an enormous thrombus of the right labia took place. I preposed to puncture it but she refused
Wilson	Mrs. John	4440	20-Apr-1869		M	first pregnancy, premature 8 months
Wilson	Mrs. Levi	3587	11-Nov-1861		F	second child
Wilson	Mrs. M. E.	2651	07-Sep-1855		M	first child
Wilson	Mrs. Richard	857	17-Jun-1843		M	third child
Wilson	Mrs. Richard	1141	19-Apr-1845		F	fourth child
Wilson	Mrs. Richard	1380	19-Jan-1847		M	fifth child
Wilson	Mrs. Richard	2008	03-Aug-1851		M	sixth child
Wilson	Mrs. Richard	2402	14-Mar-1854		F	seventh child
Wilson	Mrs. Richard	4703	10-Nov-1871		F	first pregnancy

Obstetrical Casebooks of Dr. F. E. Chatard – an alternative genealogical resource 1829-1883

Wilson	Mrs. Richard	4826	29-Mar-1873	M	second pregnancy
Wilson	Mrs. Richard C.	5074	11-Aug-1876	M	third pregnancy, "She requested to be relieved so that I gave her chloroform & applied the forceps."
Wilson	Mrs. Thomas	1764	18-Oct-1849	F	first child
Wilson	Mrs. Thomas	2032	07-Oct-1851	F	second child. Attended by Dr. Mackenzie
Wilson	Mrs. Thomas	2406	20-Mar-1854	M	third child
Wilson	Mrs. W.	183	21-Apr-1836	F	fourth child
Wilson	Mrs. W.	1309	25-Jul-1846	F	sixth child. The child was born when I arrived
Wilson	Mrs. W.	1586	19-Jun-1848	M	tenth child
Wilson	Mrs. W.	1798	22-Jan-1850	M	11th child
Wilson	Mrs. W. H.	420	20-Sep-1839	M	first child, ten pounds
Wilson	Mrs. W. H.	881	23-Aug-1843	F	fifth month
Wilson	Mrs. W. H.	1077	22-Nov-1844	F	third child, weight 11 pounds
Wilson	Mrs. W. H.	2184	29-Sep-1852	M	fifth child
Wilson	Mrs. W. W.	2222	20-Dec-1852	F	first child
Wilson	Mrs. Webster	4666	27-May-1871	F	second pregnancy
Wilson	Mrs. Webster	4868	03-Dec-1873	M	third pregnancy
Wilson	Mrs. Wm. H.	1618	20-Sep-1848	F	fourth child
Wilson	Mrs. Wm. H.	2464	17-Aug-1854	M	sixth child
Wilson	Mrs. Wm. T.	1911	08-Nov-1850	M	fourth child
Wilson	Sarah	3383	15-Jun-1860	M	colored, eighth child, child died
Winans	Mrs. Thomas	2108	02-Mar-1852	M	third child
Winans	Mrs. Thomas	2584	14-Apr-1855	F	fourth child
Winans	Mrs. Thomas	3500	14-Mar-1861	M	sixth child, premature at 5.5 months, child died at 1.5 hours, mother died 6th day.
Winans	Mrs. Wm. M.	2331	12-Sep-1853	F	first child

Obstetrical Casebooks of Dr. F. E. Chatard – an alternative genealogical resource 1829-1883

Winchester	Mrs. O.	3700	04-Nov-1862	F	second child
Winchester	Mrs. O.	3938	28-Oct-1864	M	third pregnancy
Winchester	Mrs. O. A.	3405	10-Aug-1860	M	first child
Winder	Mrs.	303	19-May-1838	F	a colored woman
Winder	Mrs. C.	141	03-Apr-1835	M	second child
Winder	Mrs. C. H.	338	30-Sep-1838	F	fourth child
Winder	Mrs. W. S.	291	18-Mar-1838	F	fifth child
Winfield	Mrs.	191	21-Jun-1836	F	sixth child, child died 40 hours after birth
Winn	Mrs.	134	28-Jan-1835	M	third child
Winn	Mrs. Frederick S.	4379	21-Oct-1868	F	first pregnancy
Winn	Mrs. J.	1435	19-May-1847	F	seventh child
Winn	Mrs. James	1142	27-Apr-1845	M	sixth child
Winn	Mrs. James	1811	10-Feb-1850	F	born 11:25 AM
Winn	Mrs. W.	278	05-Jan-1838	F	fifth child
Winn	Mrs. W.	1216	14-Oct-1845	M	third child
Winn	Mrs. William	200	13-Aug-1836	M	fourth child
Winn	Mrs. Wm.	411	27-Aug-1839	M	sixth child
Winn	Mrs. Wm.	590	25-Apr-1841	F	seventh child
Winn	Mrs. Wm.	831	11-Mar-1843	M	eighth child
Winn	Mrs. Wm.	1100	10-Jan-1845	F	ninth child
Winn	Mrs. Wm.	1509	05-Dec-1847	M	tenth child
Winn	Mrs. Wm.	1806	29-Jan-1850	F	11th child
Winn	Mrs. Wm. J.	1476	12-Sep-1847	F	fourth child
Winn	Mrs. Wm. T.	864	07-Jul-1843	F	second child
Winn (Carroll)	Mrs.	628	22-Aug-1841	F	first child

Obstetrical Casebooks of Dr. F. E. Chatard – an alternative genealogical resource 1829-1883

Wintling	Mrs.	1147	11-May-1845	M	child was born when I arrived
Withers	Mrs. W.	3788	27-Jun-1863	F	first pregnancy
Withers	Mrs. W.	3899	27-Jun-1864	M	second pregnancy
Withington	Mrs. Henry	506	30-Jun-1840	M	first child
Witridge	Mrs.	959	09-Feb-1844	F	first child
Woefflin	Mrs.	4001	10-May-1865	F	first pregnancy
Wonn	Mrs.	688	25-Feb-1842	F	fourth child
Wood	Mrs. Alexander	4369	04-Sep-1868	M	colored, first pregnancy
Wood	Mrs. Wm. H.	2384	21-Jan-1854	M	fifth child
Woodside	Mrs.	962	13-Feb-1844	F	born before 3 AM
Woodside	Mrs. Dr.	1226	07-Nov-1845	M	13th child
Woodside	Mrs. John S.	1598	05-Jul-1848	M	first child
Woodside	Mrs. John T.	1953	01-Mar-1851	M	second child
Woodside	Mrs. W. G.	2198	03-Nov-1852	M	first child
Woodside	Mrs. W. S.	3853	04-Feb-1864	F	fourth pregnancy
Woodside	Mrs. Wm. G.	3662	31-Jul-1862	M	third child
Woodside	Mrs. Wm. T.	2457	02-Aug-1854	M	second child
Woodville	Mrs. William	3027	28-Dec-1857	M	second child
Woodville, Jr.	Mrs. Wm.	2719	03-Mar-1856	F	first child. "… the child after a few gasps expired."
Woodward, Jr.	Mrs. Wm.	4491	12-Oct-1869	F	first pregnancy
Wooth	Mrs. J.	179	10-Feb-1836	M	"The child was partly born when I arrived."
Worthington	Mrs. A. C.	5223	23-Sep-1880	F	second pregnancy
Worthington	Mrs. Alexander C.	5170	06-Oct-1878	M	first pregnancy
Wright	Mrs.	613	29-Jul-1841	M	first child
Wright	Mrs. B. C.	625	17-Aug-1841	M	third child

Obstetrical Casebooks of Dr. F. E. Chatard – an alternative genealogical resource 1829-1883

Wright	Mrs. B. C.	1177	10-Jul-1845	M	fourth child
Wright	Mrs. Dr. R. C.	1106	18-Jan-1845	F	premature, four months
Wright	Mrs. J. S.	1273	15-Apr-1846	F	fourth child
Wright	Mrs. John S.	2065	04-Dec-1851	F	seventh child
Wright	Mrs. John S.	2283	16-May-1853	F	eighth child
Wright	Mrs. O. B.	2594	13-May-1855	F	sixth child
Wright	Mrs. Robert C.	810	17-Jan-1843	F	seventh child
Wright	Mrs. Robert C.	1011	05-Jul-1844	F	seventh child
Wright	Mrs. Robert C.	1467	16-Aug-1847	M	ninth child
Wright	Mrs. Robert C.	1660	08-Jan-1849	M	11th child
Wright	Mrs. Robert C.	2257	17-Mar-1853	M	12th child
Wright	Mrs. Robert C.	2542	19-Jan-1855	F	13th child
Wrinn	Mrs.	126	01-Dec-1834	M	fourth child, nine pounds
Wyatt	Mrs.	2368	16-Dec-1853	M	fourth child. "The child had several turns of the umbilical cord around its neck & life was almost extinct & was reanimated with great difficulty."
Wyeth	Mrs. C.	427	28-Oct-1839	M	sixth child
Wylie	Mrs. Samuel	5003	13-Sep-1875	F	first pregnancy
Wylie	Mrs. W.	1568	23-Apr-1848	M	first child, mother died on 11th
Wynkorp	Mrs. C. S.	3084	19-May-1858	F	second child
Wyte	Mrs. F. O.	3664	06-Aug-1862	M	fourth child
Wyte	Mrs. Major	2522	07-Dec-1854	F	second child
Wyvill	Mrs. M. D.	257		F	13th child
Wyville	Mrs. Samuel	2805	09-Oct-1856	F	first child
Wyville	Mrs. Samuel	3517	06-May-1861	F	second child

220

Obstetrical Casebooks of Dr. F. E. Chatard – an alternative genealogical resource 1829-1883

Yeates	Mrs. Dr. J. L.	1890	16-Sep-1850	M	premature labor, sixth child
Yellott	Mrs. Coleman	2644	24-Aug-1855	M	third child
Young	Mrs.	1944	04-Feb-1851	F	fifth child, premature 7 months
Young	Mrs. Alexander	1156	21-May-1845	F	first child. She died on the ninth day of puerperal fever
Zimmer	Mrs.	361	30-Jan-1839	M	born 9:15 PM

221

www.ingramcontent.com/pod-product-compliance
Lightning Source LLC
Chambersburg PA
CBHW050138170426
43197CB00011B/1882